# Praise for

# WALKING BROOKLYN

**"Adrienne's *Walking Brooklyn* is the best type of animated inanimate guide. It made me chuckle & made me learn! Bravissimo!"**

—Native-born Brooklynite and licensed NYC Tour Guide
Matt Levy, The Levys' Unique New York!

**"Easy to follow tours for an easy to love city. *Walking Brooklyn* offers insider secrets to getting to know the best of Brooklyn. Adrienne Onofri makes you an honorary Brooklynite with her fact-packed guide of this dynamic and beloved city."**

—Wendy Zarganis, About.com Guide to Brooklyn

**"Great . . . well-written and informative."**
—Ruth Edebohls, Coordinator of Urban Tours,
Brooklyn Center for the Urban Environment

**"*Walking Brooklyn* is a must for avid explorers wishing to truly understand and travel around Brooklyn."**

—Art and Susan Zuckerman, Z Travel and Leisure Tours;
Hosts *Z Travel and Leisure* WVOX Radio

D1275514

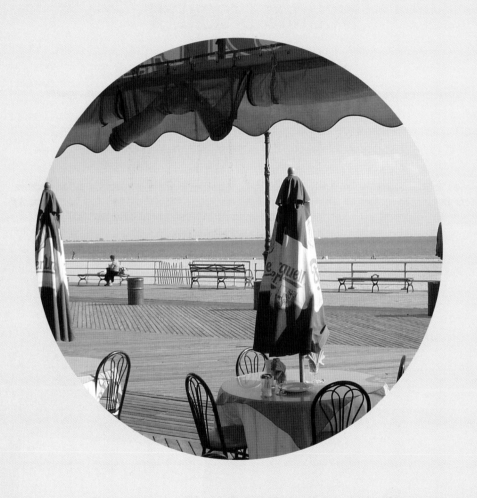

# WALKING BROOKLYN

### 30 tours exploring
### historical legacies,
### neighborhood culture,
### side streets, and waterways

Adrienne Onofri

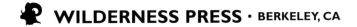

**WILDERNESS PRESS** · BERKELEY, CA

Walking Brooklyn: 30 tours exploring historical legacies, neighborhood culture, side streets, and waterways

**1st EDITION June 2007**

Copyright © 2007 by Adrienne Onofri

Cover photos copyright © 2007 by Adrienne Onofri, except for following: Mathew Grimm (front, bottom center) and Dana Sommers (front, middle left; back, top right; and back, bottom right)
Interior photos © 2007 by Adrienne Onofri, except for following: Mathew Grimm (pp. 5 and 201) and Dana Sommers (pp. 75, 81, and 85)
Maps: Bart Wright/Lohnes + Wright
Book and cover design: Larry B. Van Dyke
Book editor: Julie Van Pelt
Layout: Lisa Pletka

ISBN 978-0-89997-430-9
UPC 7-19609-97430-7

Manufactured in China

Published by:  **Wilderness Press**
               **1200 5th Street**
               **Berkeley, CA 94710**
               **(800) 443-7227; FAX (510) 558-1696**
               **info@wildernesspress.com**
               **www.wildernesspress.com**
Visit our website for a complete listing of our books and for ordering information.

*Cover photos:*   *Front, clockwise from bottom center:* Brooklyn Bridge; Russian Orthodox Cathedral of the Transfiguration of Our Lord; M&I International grocery store in Brighton Beach; Prospect Park's Vale of Cashmere; Coney Island; St. John's Place in Park Slope; Sheepshead Bay. *Back, clockwise from bottom left:* Clam shucker at Randazzo's in Sheepshead Bay; the Soldiers' and Sailors' Memorial Arch in Grand Army Plaza; and Prospect Park in fall.
*Frontispiece:*   The Boardwalk in Brighton Beach.

**SAFETY NOTICE:** Although Wilderness Press and the author have made every attempt to ensure that the information in this book is accurate at press time, they are not responsible for any loss, damage, injury, or inconvenience that may occur to anyone while using this book. You are responsible for your own safety and health while following the walking trips described here. Always check local conditions, know your own limitations, and consult a map.

# acknowledgments

I want to thank Wilderness Press and the people there who have guided and supported me. As this is my first book, I needed their assistance! Thanks also to Ted Botha, who brought me and Wilderness Press together. I also thank everyone in Brooklyn who provided insights and answers as I was roaming: park rangers, historians, shopkeepers, restaurateurs, staff at historic and cultural sites, and folks from the Brooklyn Chamber of Commerce, Brooklyn Historical Society, Brooklyn Tourism and Visitors Center, and Brooklyn Center for the Urban Environment, as well as the inquisitive, informative residents I met on the streets.

I could not have written a book like this without my parents, since they are the ones who taught me walk, to enjoy walking as a pastime, and to love New York City. Finally, I would like to salute all the people who have helped shape the land and lore of Brooklyn, making it such a vibrant, important place—from Frederick Law Olmsted to Jackie Robinson, Lady Deborah Moody to Emily Roebling, and many others over the last 350 years. Brooklyn's citizenry and visitors are forever in your debt.

# author's note

Every guidebook must bear the warning that its information is subject to change, but that may be an understatement for a book about Brooklyn. Things are changing so much that while working on this book I'd return to a place I had visited a couple of weeks earlier to find it cordoned off for renovation or remodeling. Or I'd go back to some place that had been hidden under scaffolding to find a striking new building or beautifully rehabilitated old one.

I have done my best to verify that this book is up-to-date and to make note of where change may occur by the time you take a Brooklyn walk. But redevelopments, demolitions, and new construction are continually being proposed, announced, challenged, or begun, so some things could look a little different from what I've described. A $4 billion, 22-acre project that would profoundly alter Brooklyn's skyline and streetscape hangs in the balance as I write this. That planned rehab of the old Atlantic Yards rail depot at Flatbush and Atlantic Aves. includes a pro basketball arena, more than a dozen residential high-rises, and a Frank Gehry skyscraper. Though the plan has received almost all necessary government approvals, fervent opposition persists, including a star-studded protest group called Develop Don't Destroy Brooklyn.

Another caveat that comes with any city guidebook is the reminder that you are indeed in a city, so exercise common sense: be alert and cautious (but not scared!), and enjoy these walks during the daytime.

And some practical pointers for taking these walks: Pick up a Brooklyn bus map (free at most subway stations) so that if you want to cut a walk short you can find the nearest bus or subway. To see the inside of Brooklyn's churches—the borough is known as the "city of churches"—plan your walks around scheduled services, the only time when churches are usually open.

This book has not only been a professional venture but has also fulfilled a personal quest. I was three blocks from the World Trade Center on the morning of 9/11 and continued working in the neighborhood that fall, when armed military personnel were posted at every corner and the odor from the smoldering wreckage permeated the area. That the city is once again teeming with activity is a testament to that most laudable human quality: resilience. I have wanted to do something to express my affection for New York and my pride in its recovery. Writing a book that encourages people to explore and appreciate the city turned out to be that thing.

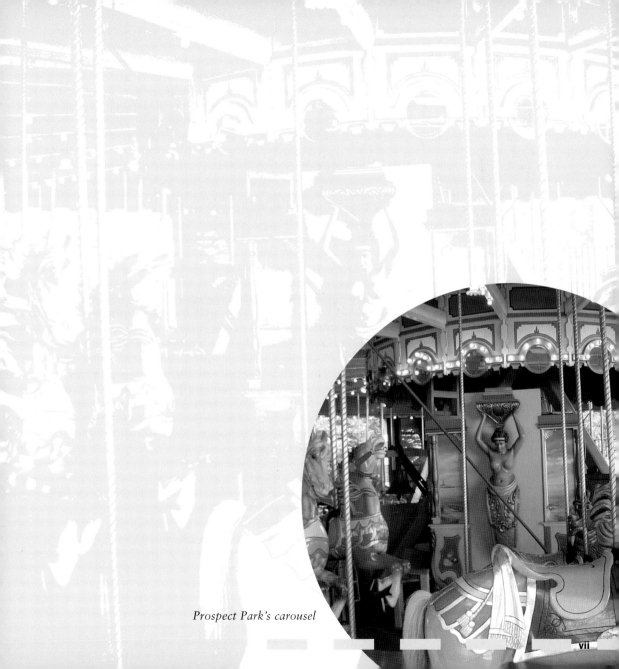

*Prospect Park's carousel*

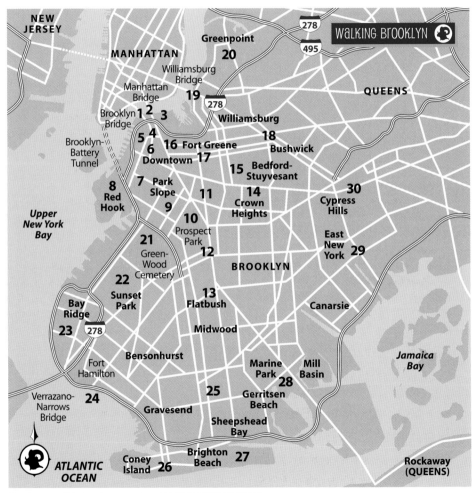

NEW JERSEY

MANHATTAN

Greenpoint
**20**

Williamsburg Bridge

Manhattan Bridge
**19**

278

Brooklyn Bridge
**1 2 3**

Williamsburg

**18**

Brooklyn-Battery Tunnel

**5 4**
**6 16** Fort Greene
**17**
Downtown

Bushwick

**15** Bedford-Stuyvesant

**8**
Red Hook

**7 Park Slope**

**11**

**14**
Crown Heights

**30**
Cypress Hills

**9**

**10**
Prospect Park

East New York **29**

Upper New York Bay

**21**
Green-Wood Cemetery

**12**

BROOKLYN

**22**
Sunset Park

**13**
Flatbush

Canarsie

Bay Ridge
**23** 278

Midwood

Fort Hamilton

Bensonhurst

Marine Park **28**

Mill Basin

Jamaica Bay

Verrazano-Narrows Bridge
**24**

Gravesend

**25**

Gerritsen Beach

Sheepshead Bay

ATLANTIC OCEAN

Coney Island **26**

Brighton Beach **27**

Rockaway (QUEENS)

QUEENS

WALKING BROOKLYN

278

495

Numbers on this locator map correspond to Walk numbers.

# TABLE OF CONTENTS

# INTRODUCTION

Sometimes it seems like all of Brooklyn should be coated in sepia tones, so strong is the nostalgia surrounding it. To those who grew up or raised a family here in the 1930s, '40s, or '50s, Brooklyn is the land of stickball and egg creams, Old World relatives, Ebbets Field and the Loews and RKO movie palaces, the Parachute Jump and Shoot the Chutes rides at the beach . . . and of an accent that pronounces *oi* as *er* and vice versa (this accent is said to have originated in the neighborhood of *Greenpernt*).

Then there is 21st-century Brooklyn—artsy and cool, already dubbed the new Manhattan, and already incurring a backlash for it. Young people, families with small children, and Manhattan exiles who desire more room inside their homes and less crowding outside have been repopulating once-neglected neighborhoods, rediscovering the riverfront and old industrial lots, and opening art galleries, performance spaces, funky bars and coffeehouses, and trendy boutiques.

While this renaissance has renewed hometown pride in Brooklyn, there is a disconnect between today's Brooklyn and the Brooklyn of so many cherished memories. Many of the newer Brooklynites grew up far from Kings County. They may not even know they're supposed to hate Walter O'Malley for banishing the Dodgers to California, or Robert Moses for bulldozing a highway through their streets. And so we have a place defined by both the past and the future, a personality both nostalgic and on the cutting edge.

Of course, many other events have left their mark on Brooklyn—the devastating assault by the king's army during the Revolutionary War, the high-bourgeois Victorian age, the lurid decline of the 1970s, to name just a few. Brooklyn has the unique history of having been an independent city and before that several different cities and townships. It also boasts of the great outdoors, with three parks of 450-plus acres and a shoreline that stretches from river to bay to ocean.

With all this diversity in its history, its geography, its very essence, Brooklyn is a most exciting place to explore up close and personal . . . the kind of exploring done best on foot. This book provides routes to follow and identifies points of interest, but you will set your own pace and make your own discoveries as you walk, choosing perhaps to spend time inside some place along the way or even veer off-course to see more of something that catches your fancy. You're in the most walkable of cities, so get some comfortable shoes and have fun!

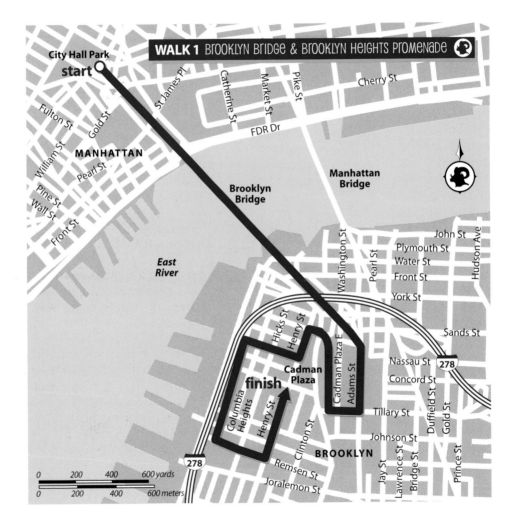

**WALK 1** Brooklyn Bridge & Brooklyn Heights Promenade

# 1 BrookLyN Bridge aND BrookLyN Heights PromeNade: riverside rambles

BOUNDARIES: **Park Row/Centre St. (Manhattan), Adams St., Remsen St., Promenade**
DISTANCE: **Approx. 2¼ miles**
SUBWAY: **4, 5, or 6 to Brooklyn Bridge**

"What a lovely view from, heaven looks at you from, the Brooklyn Bridge," sang Frank Sinatra in the 1947 film *It Happened in Brooklyn*. There are other ways to enter Brooklyn, but none is as famous (or as scenic) as the Brooklyn Bridge. It is, in fact, one of the most famous bridges in the world—an engineering marvel when it was built 120-plus years ago and still one of America's architectural masterworks. After crossing the bridge, you'll stroll through part of Brooklyn Heights and then take another riverside walk, on the Brooklyn Heights Promenade. This trip may be the ultimate New York City photo op, as it offers views of virtually all of the city's most recognizable landmarks.

● **Begin in Manhattan. Pedestrians get onto the bridge from Park Row/Centre St., next to the Municipal Building. Manhattan sights visible from the small plaza there include the domed and somewhat dwarfed City Hall and, beyond it, the Gothic-inspired Woolworth Building, tallest in the world from 1913 to 1930.**

● **The Brooklyn Bridge was itself the tallest structure in the city—and the world's longest (1,595 feet) suspension bridge—when it opened in May 1883, linking Manhattan and what was then the separate city of Brooklyn. On your way up to the bridge, look to your right at what was once the world's tallest building (now bearing the Trump name) at 40 Wall St.—there's a spire extending from its pyramidal top. Originally known as the Bank of Manhattan, it was constructed at the same time as the Chrysler Building, and the two architects—former partners—were competing to build the world's highest skyscraper. The Bank of Manhattan opened first in 1930, but then a secretly planned 185-foot spire was put atop the Chrysler Building, ending 40 Wall St.'s reign after just a few weeks.**

- The bridge officially begins where the concrete ramp gives way to wooden planks. As directed by signs, stay in the right (south) lane when walking on the vehicle-free upper level; the left lane is for bicyclists. There are benches on the bridge, so you can make this walk as leisurely as you like.

- When you reach the bridge's first tower, to the south you'll be able to see Governors Island (home to a shuttered Coast Guard facility) and South Street Seaport, with its antique sailing ships, as well as the Chrysler and Met Life buildings to the northwest. That busy highway at the river's edge is the FDR Drive, which carries upward of 150,000 cars a day.

- Around the tower, a series of engraved plaques explain the bridge's construction step-by-step. Caissons—huge airtight chambers installed in the riverbed so men could work underwater laying the foundations—were a major innovation, though 20 workers died from decompression sickness (the bends). Just past the tower another group of plaques identify some of the Brooklyn sights and describe a bit of the borough's and bridge's history.

- As you continue along the boardwalk between the towers, you'll have a full view of the Manhattan Bridge and will start to see the Williamsburg Bridge behind it. These two spans, opened in 1909 and 1903, respectively, have neither the iconic status nor aesthetic cachet of the Brooklyn Bridge, but the three together create a striking image and apt symbol of this city that's always on the move. You also now have a terrific view of the Midtown skyline—dominated by the Empire State Building—and the Statue of Liberty comes into view on your right once you're past the bridge's midpoint. This platform was the world's highest human-made observatory when the bridge opened.

- More informational plaques around the bridge's second tower identify the Manhattan sights and describe the East River bridges and islands as well as some of the significant vessels that have plied these waters over time. A plaque on the tower honors Emily Roebling, who supervised construction after her husband, engineer Washington Roebling, was paralyzed with the bends (his father, John, designed the bridge, but died before construction began).

● Take one last look back at the awe-inspiring views from this awe-inspiring bridge before stepping off the wooden planks and back onto pavement (the "off-ramp"). To the right you start to see some of the charming brickfronts of Brooklyn Heights.

● Go to the right when the pedestrian lanes diverge, near where a large green-and-white WELCOME TO BROOKLYN road sign comes into view. The sign also says HOW SWEET IT IS!—the catchphrase of Brooklyn-born TV legend Jackie Gleason. On your way down the off-ramp, you'll see a grassy knoll with benches to your right. This is Walt Whitman Park, one of many places in Brooklyn named after the world-renowned poet who lived and worked in the borough (and penned verses about it). Ahead of you are the glassy office buildings of Downtown Brooklyn. The footpath runs along Adams St., aka Brooklyn Bridge Blvd., and as you reach the end you're reunited with vehicular traffic.

● Turn right on Tillary St. and proceed one block to Cadman Plaza Park, which separates Downtown Brooklyn and Brooklyn Heights. The 10-acre park is named for Samuel Cadman, a Congregationalist pastor in Brooklyn for 36 years and one of the first radio preachers. The park contains a memorial to Brooklyn's World War II veterans, flanked by 24-foot-tall statues (the man represents the battlefield; the woman, home and hearth). Walk north through the park—past the war memorial, down the steps, and toward the bust of former New York mayor William Jay Gaynor. Exit the park to your left when you're looking at Gaynor.

● Cross Cadman Plaza W. and walk on Middagh St. one block to Henry St. On your right is the old factory of Peaks Mason Mints, a candy maker

*Brooklyn Bridge*

based here from 1892 to 1949; some of their treats are today produced by the Tootsie Roll company. On your left is the current office of the *Brooklyn Daily Eagle*. The *Brooklyn Eagle* was one of the newspapers that employed a young journalist named Walt Whitman in the 1840s, but the current incarnation is a different paper that revived the name.

● Turn left on Henry, a good place to refresh with a snack—perhaps a bakery treat from Cranberry's or, farther along, an ice cream at the Blue Pig.

● Turn right on Orange St. See the Brooklyn Heights walk for most of the area's sight-seeing, but we can't pass up the Plymouth Church of the Pilgrims on your right. Congregationalist minister Henry Ward Beecher, brother of *Uncle Tom's Cabin* author Harriet Beecher Stowe, preached here from 1849 to 1887. He was a leading progressive and huge celebrity in his day (complete with his own tabloidy adultery scandal). Other prominent social activists have also spoken here, among them Charles Dickens, Clara Barton, Mark Twain, and Martin Luther King, Jr. The church's gorgeous stained glass portrays secular historical scenes, mostly revolving around the idea of liberty, and includes five windows by Tiffany. In the garden are a statue of Beecher (holding one of his mock slave auctions that essentially bought the slave's freedom) and a bas-relief of Abraham Lincoln, who worshipped at the church; both were sculpted by Mount Rushmore carver Gutzon Borglum.

● Cross the street named Columbia Heights to get onto the Brooklyn Heights Promenade. Two of the Jehovah's Witnesses' many residences in Brooklyn Heights sit across from each other at the Orange St./Columbia Heights intersection. The unsightly one on your left has no real history, but the Margaret on your right is named after the grand hotel that stood here from 1889 until it burned down in 1980. Betty Smith wrote *A Tree Grows in Brooklyn* while living at the Margaret. Emily and Washington Roebling lived in a now-demolished house on this block of Columbia Heights while the Brooklyn Bridge was being erected. Washington, bedridden with the bends—or a nervous breakdown, according to some historians—watched construction through a telescope. Poet Hart Crane later lived in the house while he penned his epic poem "The Bridge."

- Check out the little pocket park, centered on a zodiac-themed sculpture, at this end of the Promenade, then enjoy your walk and the spectacular views of Lower Manhattan, the Brooklyn Bridge, and the Statue of Liberty. You'll quickly understand why the Esplanade (as some call it) is beloved of photographers, canoodlers, and dog walkers alike.

- At Clark St., the second street after Orange connecting to the Promenade, is the former site of Fort Stirling, built by American forces in March 1776 but seized by the British that summer in the Battle of Brooklyn. Americans regained the fort in 1783 but razed it because of the taint of British occupation.

- As lovely as it is, the Promenade is also a bittersweet spot, as it had provided an unparalleled view of the Twin Towers. A framed black-and-white photograph of the pre-9/11 view is affixed to the Promenade railing at Pierrepont St. (the street after Clark). Farther on, a historic marker on a boulder where Montague St. meets the Promenade notes the approximate location of George Washington's headquarters during his troops' retreat after the disastrous Battle of Brooklyn.

- At the south end of the Promenade, at Remsen St., a plaque shows the 1873 view. Today's view includes the Verrazano-Narrows Bridge (the country's longest suspension bridge, which connects Brooklyn and Staten Island).

- Walk on Remsen to Henry and turn left. Our Lady of Lebanon Maronite Catholic Cathedral at this intersection was built in 1846 for the Congregationalist Plymouth Church, which moved into the Church of the Pilgrims over on Orange when they merged about 100 years later. Walk on Henry to Clark for the 2 or 3 subway.

## POINTS OF INTEREST

**Cadman Plaza Park** Tillary St. and Cadman Plaza, Brooklyn, NY 11201
**Cranberry's** 48 Henry St., Brooklyn, NY 11201, 718-624-3500
**The Blue Pig** 60 Henry St., Brooklyn, NY 11201, 718-596-6301

## route summary

1. Begin at Manhattan terminus of Brooklyn Bridge.
2. Cross Brooklyn Bridge.
3. Turn right on Tillary St.
4. Cross Cadman Plaza Park.
5. Turn left on Middagh St.
6. Turn left on Henry St.
7. Turn right on Orange St.
8. Walk the length of the Brooklyn Heights Promenade.
9. Turn left on Remsen St.
10. Turn left on Henry and get the subway at Clark St.

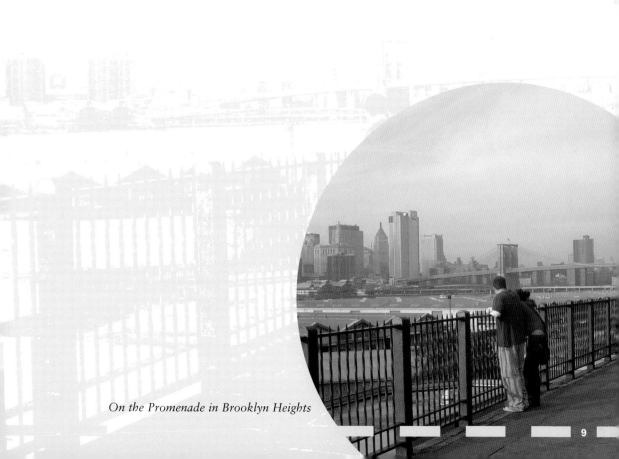

*On the Promenade in Brooklyn Heights*

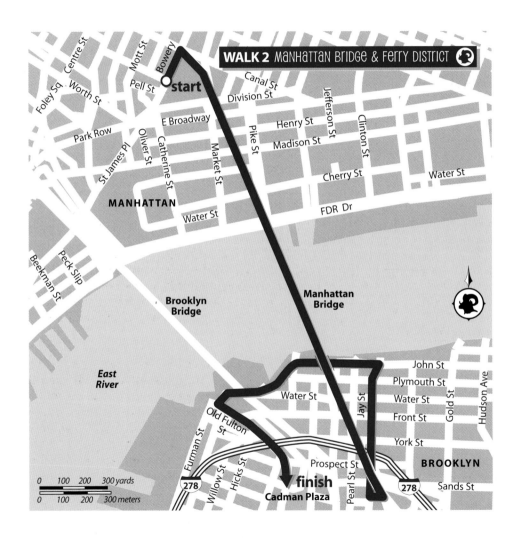

WALK 2 Manhattan Bridge & Ferry District

MANHATTAN

Centre St
Mott St
Bowery
Pell St
Foley Sq
Worth St
Park Row
St James Pl
Oliver St
Catherine St
Market St
E Broadway
Canal St
Division St
Pike St
Henry St
Madison St
Jefferson St
Clinton St
Cherry St
Water St
Water St
FDR Dr
Water St

**start**

Beekman St
Peck Slip

**Brooklyn Bridge**

**Manhattan Bridge**

East River

Furman St
Willow St
Hicks St
Old Fulton St
Water St
Jay St
Water St
Front St
York St
Prospect St
Pearl St
John St
Plymouth St
Gold St
Hudson Ave
Sands St

**BROOKLYN**

**finish**
**Cadman Plaza**

278
278

0   100   200   300 yards
0   100   200   300 meters

# 2 Manhattan Bridge and Ferry District: Vital Links Across the River

**BOUNDARIES:** **Bowery (Manhattan), Jay St., Sands St., Water St.**
**DISTANCE:** **Approx. 2½ miles**
**SUBWAY:** **N, R, or 6 to Canal St. (Lafayette St. exit)**

The 1,470-foot-long Manhattan Bridge is the youngest of the three lower East River spans, completed in 1909. Overshadowed in historical significance and renown by its southern neighbor, the Brooklyn Bridge, it gets only a fraction of that bridge's pedestrian traffic. The Manhattan Bridge footpath, in fact, just reopened in 2001 after a 40-plus-year closure. On this walk, you reach Brooklyn via the Manhattan Bridge, get a glimpse of the up-and-coming Dumbo neighborhood as you head to the water's edge, and then follow the river through the Ferry District and wind up beneath the Brooklyn Bridge.

● Begin in Manhattan on the Bowery at Bayard St., one block south of Canal St., in the heart of Chinatown. Note the Mahayana Buddhist Temple on the far side of Canal St. and the exquisite HSBC building (a worldwide bank with Chinese origins) across the Bowery. Walk up the sidewalk on the east side of the Bowery, which soon becomes the pedestrian lane of the Manhattan Bridge.

● The Manhattan Bridge has the most grandiose entrance of any New York City bridge. Its massive arch was modeled after Paris's Porte St. Denis, its colonnade after the one by Bernini at St. Peter's in Rome. The frieze above the arch depicts a frontier scene, while sculptures beside it represent commerce and industry. The first spectacular view of the Brooklyn Bridge and Lower Manhattan skyline comes when you're directly over the highway (the FDR Drive). Picture taking may be impeded by the chain-link fence that encloses the pedestrian lane, but don't fret—this view will be unobstructed from several spots along the walk in Brooklyn.

● On the crossing, one of the most noticeable buildings on the Brooklyn side is Dumbo's Clocktower Building, which you'll be in front of later. As you near the end of the bridge, the handiwork of Robert Moses dominates the view: the Brooklyn-Queens

Expressway, or BQE—one of many road projects shepherded (some would say ramrodded) into existence by the omnipotent public-works chief Moses, whose highways redefined (some would say devastated) several Brooklyn neighborhoods.

● After walking down the steps from the bridge, go to the right on Jay St. and enter Dumbo—down under the Manhattan Bridge overpass—a turn-of-the-century industrial hub revived in the past decade by artists and entrepreneurs. The high-rise in front of you across Jay is 90 Sands St., where approximately 1,000 Jehovah's Witnesses live, and their Watchtower Society is headquartered in the area. Carson McCullers, the Georgia-born novelist of *The Heart Is a Lonely Hunter* fame, wrote about "vivacious" Sands St.—"where sailors spend their evenings when they come here to port"—in a 1941 essay "Brooklyn Is My Neighborhood." That was a polite way of alluding to all the bars and brothels. Sands lost that identity when waterfront commerce diminished.

● Cross Sands, and at Prospect St. walk diagonally beneath the bridge to continue on Jay. At 85 Jay St., the tract of land on your right past York St., stood P.S. 7, a 120-year-old school listed on the National Register of Historic Places but razed in 1992 to make way for the Jehovah's Witnesses' largest residential complex. Across the street is development more typical of Dumbo's rejuvenation: the brand-new superluxe J Condominium.

● Jay is one of Dumbo's main streets for trendy retailers, most with an art and design slant. Ben Forman & Sons' former metalworking plant at Water St. has become the Jay Street Arts Building. Several stores selling custom-crafted, exotic, or vintage furniture are located between Front and Plymouth Sts. The tracks between Water and Plymouth were not for public trolleys but rather cargo transport for neighborhood industry around the turn of the century.

● At John St., turn left and proceed to Adams St., where you enter Brooklyn Bridge Park. This city park opened in 2003 and is supposed to eventually extend 1⅓ miles to Atlantic Ave. on the other side of the Brooklyn Bridge. Take the shorefront path, passing under the Manhattan Bridge. You'll come to a small semicircular plot jutting into the water—a picture-perfect spot for a photograph of the Brooklyn Bridge and Manhattan.

- Keep walking along the water to a cove and its stone-covered beach. In nice weather the water looks almost tempting, but of course this is the notorious East River. Though it has been cleaned over the last three decades, swimming is still discouraged except for a few charity swims each year. You can see the Empire State Building from the cove. Continue in the direction of the Brooklyn Bridge and exit the park at Plymouth and Main St. The Clocktower Building you saw from the bridge is to your left.

- Rising above you on the right are the immense Empire Stores, a Civil War–era coffee warehouse. The brick exterior is speckled with iron stars—an ornamental flourish around the support beams that run through the building—and you can still make out some of the words painted on the Main St. side. Plans are underway to renovate and fill the interior with a marketplace of art galleries and cafés by 2015.

- Enter Empire-Fulton Ferry State Park beneath the warehouse. The park, due to be incorporated into Brooklyn Bridge Park as that city park grows, was developed around a natural cove. You'll pass a few huge old anchorages in the park, and if you follow the wooden boardwalk to the end you'll see the Statue of Liberty. Backtrack on the path, or walk across the grass if it's allowed, and when you're facing the Empire Stores, go to the right. Then turn left to exit the park. There are public restrooms and a visitor information office inside the Empire Stores building. The topless brick building on your right was a tobacco inspection warehouse; it's now used for private and public special events.

- Turn right onto Water and follow it up to Old Fulton St. On your right is

*Old Fulton St.*

the Fulton Ferry Landing, just beside the Brooklyn Bridge. In 1776, George Washington massed 9,500 troops here for a furtive evacuation across a river filled with British warships. The Americans had just been routed in the Battle of Brooklyn, and the retreat prevented complete defeat and therefore saved the fledgling nation. In 1814, Robert Fulton launched the first steamboat from here, opening up travel between Brooklyn and Manhattan. Plaques on the restored pier commemorate this history, and the metal railing around the pier features section nine of Walt Whitman's poem "Crossing Brooklyn Ferry."

● At the corner of Water and Old Fulton, you can dine on delicious Italian specialties at Pete's Downtown with the same fantastic view—but far more affordable pricing—as the prestigious River Café across the street. Owned by a fourth-generation Brooklyn restaurateur, Pete's occupies an 1835 building that started out as a hotel. A couple of other NYC eating institutions are at the ferry landing. The Brooklyn Ice Cream Factory opened in the old fireboat house in 2001 and offers eight basic flavors (all made on the premises); some have already anointed it as the city's best ice cream. You can pair it

## DOCKED AT THE LANDING: BARGEMUSIC

Classical music is performed by world-class artists year-round inside a barge permanently moored at the Fulton Ferry Landing. Bargemusic recently embarked on its fourth decade of chamber-music concerts. Some love it for the view—from the front rows, all of Lower Manhattan and the South Street Seaport twinkles before you. Some love it for the intimacy—a cozy, wood-paneled room where you can chat with the musicians at intermission and help yourself to wine and cheese or coffee and a sweet (donations appreciated). Some love it for the extraordinary sensation of rocking softly as the music plays. And many love Bargemusic for the music itself—piano and string pieces, ranging from premieres to the canon, performed by musicians from around the globe. Bargemusic was founded by violinist Olga Bloom, who still attends concerts, which are held Thursday, Friday, and Saturday evenings and Sunday afternoons. There's a free concert one Saturday afternoon per month. Whatever time you choose to attend, two things are guaranteed: a simultaneous dazzling of the senses and the yen to return.

with what's often called the city's best pizza at Grimaldi's, located a few storefronts to the left on Old Fulton.

● Across from Grimaldi's stands the fortresslike Eagle Warehouse & Storage Company. It was named after the *Brooklyn Eagle* newspaper that occupied the site prior to the warehouse's construction in 1892, and that from 1846 to 1848 employed a crusading journalist named Walt Whitman. The red-brick building now contains—what else?—luxury apartments.

● As you walk up Old Fulton, note the white building at 1 Front St. on your left. It was built in 1869 for the Long Island Safe Deposit Company, which stayed only till 1891; since then it's been a warehouse and then a succession of bars and restaurants. Next to it, the Greek Revival building at 5–7 Front St. dates to 1834 and is considered the city's oldest surviving office building.

● Stay on Old Fulton as it curves around to the right, crossing Hicks and Henry Sts., and becomes Cadman Plaza W. Just past Middagh St. is the High St. station, where you can take the A or C subway.

## POINTS OF INTEREST

**Brooklyn Bridge Park** Plymouth St. between Adams and Main Sts., Brooklyn, NY 11201, 718-802-0603

**Empire-Fulton Ferry State Park** 6 New Dock St., Brooklyn, NY 11201, 718-858-4708

**Pete's Downtown** 2 Water St., Brooklyn, NY 11201, 718-858-3510

**Brooklyn Ice Cream Factory** Fulton Ferry Landing, Brooklyn, NY 11201, 718-246-3963

**Grimaldi's** 19 Old Fulton St., Brooklyn, NY 11201, 718-858-4300

**Bargemusic** Fulton Ferry Landing, Brooklyn, NY 11201, 718-624-4061/2083

# route summary

1.  Begin at Manhattan entrance to Manhattan Bridge.
2.  Cross Manhattan Bridge.
3.  Turn right on Jay St.
4.  Go left on John St. to Adams St.
5.  Walk through Brooklyn Bridge Park and adjacent Empire-Fulton Ferry State Park.
6.  Turn right on Water St. to Fulton Ferry Landing.
7.  Turn left on Old Fulton St.
8.  Bear right as Old Fulton becomes Cadman Plaza W. and proceed to Middagh St. for the subway.

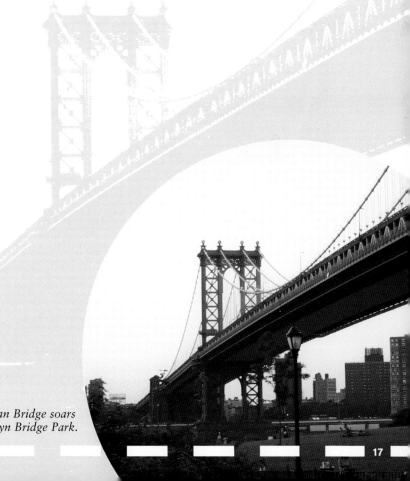

*The Manhattan Bridge soars above Brooklyn Bridge Park.*

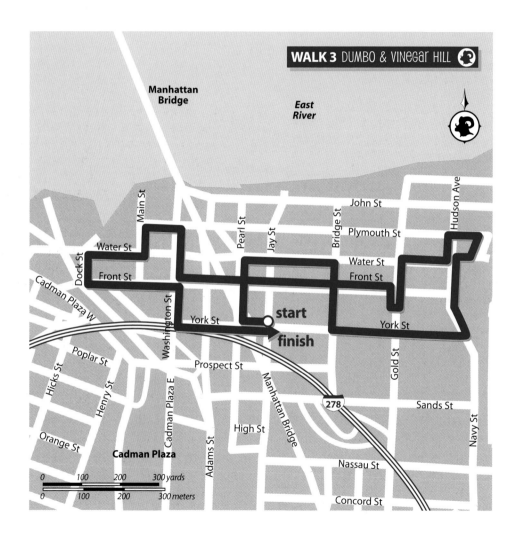

Manhattan
Bridge

East
River

Main St

Water St

Front St

Dock St

Cadman Plaza W

Washington St

York St

Poplar St

Hicks St

Henry St

Orange St

**Cadman Plaza**

Cadman Plaza E

Adams St

Prospect St

High St

Manhattan Bridge

278

Nassau St

Concord St

Sands St

Navy St

Gold St

York St

Front St

Water St

Plymouth St

John St

Bridge St

Hudson Ave

Pearl St

Jay St

**start**

**finish**

0      100      200      300 yards
0      100      200      300 meters

# 3 DUMBO AND VINEGAR HILL: BIG-BUCKS BOHEMIA

**BOUNDARIES:** **York St., Little St., Plymouth St., Dock St.**
**DISTANCE:** **Approx. 2¼ miles**
**SUBWAY:** **F to York St.**

In the past decade, artists and dot-commers have turned this no-man's-land down under the Manhattan Bridge overpass into another Soho, converting warehouses into trendy residential and cultural venues. The attitude may be bohemian, but the real-estate prices certainly aren't: prime units in new luxury condo buildings go for upward of a million bucks. But the views— arguably Dumbo's greatest asset—are priceless. Near the river and from the upper stories of buildings, there are sweeping vistas of Lower Manhattan and its three bridges, while snippets of them peek through open spaces in the streets of Dumbo. This walk takes you through those streets and into adjacent Vinegar Hill, an oft-overlooked enclave.

- You'll be on Jay St. when you come out of the subway station. Since part of Dumbo's appeal is its authentic old-fashioned stone streets, turn left onto York St., which hasn't been paved over. This will also make you truly dumbo (no offense) in Dumbo: as you approach Pearl St., you'll be right under the bridge overpass.

- Turn right and head downhill on Pearl for a unique experience: walking amid the arches supporting a bridge that carries about 80,000 vehicles a day. The view ahead of the Empire State Building may make you think you're facing west, since Manhattan is on the west side of the river. But both this corner of Brooklyn and the area of Manhattan opposite jut out from their respective islands, so in Dumbo, toward the river is north.

- Two of Dumbo's offbeat enterprises are on the block of Pearl north of Front St. On your right, you'll come first to Jan Larsen Art, a gallery with a stereo and lounge space for enjoying "sonic craft." A couple of doors down is Halcyon, a record store catering to deejays that also hosts art exhibits and features indoor landscaping—an Astroturf floor, two mini-rock gardens with paths, and seats for sampling the music in comfort.

- Turn right on Water St. Journey, a home-décor boutique, is on your right. Then you cross Jay and pass a couple of old brick warehouses, followed by the pastel-colored buildings once occupied by Kirkman & Son, a manufacturer of laundry and dish detergent established in 1831 (and eventually merged into Colgate-Palmolive).

- Turn right on Bridge St. and walk two blocks. Back at York, you'll be in front of a 1909 factory building most noticeable for the glazed terra cotta ornamentation toward the top, including shields bearing the letters TM at the corners. That stood for Thomson Meter, but the building is identified more with another former corporate tenant: Eskimo Pies.

- Turn left on York. On your right is Farragut, a public-housing complex that stretches across two blocks in each direction. Past Gold St. on your left, an angel and the Virgin Mary smile down upon you from the stately but abandoned St. George's Church, constructed in 1914 but not used since 2003. Neighborhood preservationists fear it may meet the same fate as the early-1800s house next door, which was demolished in 2004 after being left to decay.

- At Navy St., if you were to go to the right, you'd find yourself at the birthplace of Al Capone (95 Navy St.). But to explore Vinegar Hill, turn left on Navy, which soon becomes Hudson Ave. Hudson is the main drag of Vinegar Hill, but without a main drag's typical traffic. In fact, Vinegar Hill almost seems misplaced: it's a 19th-century village scrunched between such modern structures as a housing project and a power plant. The neighborhood, named after a battle of Irish independence, had a largely Irish population throughout the 1800s. After the turn of the century, Lithuanians started to move in, and by 1930 they constituted three-quarters of the population (the bricked-up church on York St. served Lithuanians).

- At Front St., you'll pass the old Boorum & Pease warehouse on your left and an upscale 21st-century apartment building opposite it at 85 Hudson Ave. The house at 79 Hudson Ave., with dark wood doors, is at least 130 years old. How do you know the BUTCHER SHOP signage at 72 Hudson Ave. is fake? There are no shops in Vinegar Hill; that was painted on the windows for a TV commercial. The rectangular stones with which the street is still paved are known as Belgian blocks, and these on Hudson are originals from around 1860.

- Turn right on Evans St., which ends at Little St., abutting the decommissioned but once mightily important Brooklyn Navy Yard. To your right on Little is the house built in 1806 for the Navy Yard commandant—a Hamptons-like estate designed by the same architect as the U.S. Capitol. Vinegar Hill itself was something of a red-light district during the Navy Yard's heyday, earning the nickname Hell's Half Acre.

- Go to the left on Little, then left on Plymouth St., and left a third time on Hudson. Original ownership of the corner house (#49), which may have been built as early as 1801, has been traced to the family of Vinegar Hill founder John Jackson. Storefronts line this street, but there are no longer stores inside; they are residences or studios. The disappearing BARBER SHOP etched on the window at #51 is left over from a long-ago shuttered business.

- Turn right on Water, then left on Gold, with a row of brick Greek Revival houses—#69 to #75—from the 1840s.

- Cross Front St. The property enclosed by a yellow fence used to be a gas station and now belongs to Dorje Ling Buddhist Center. Look into the lot at the temple's colorful doorway, statuary, huge tent, and prayer flags suspended like a car dealership's plastic banners. Residences on this block include modern apartments as well as homes at #100 and #102 dating to the early 1800s.

- Backtrack to Front and turn left. A mid-1800s church was razed in 1992 and replaced with the parking lot on your right. Local furor over the demolition led to Vinegar Hill's designation as a historic district, which protects buildings. Some of the neighborhood's oldest rowhouses,

*The Eskimo Pie building*

circa 1845, survive at #237 to #249. The tall building at #231–233, originally owned by Benjamin Moore Paint Company, dates to 1908 and was the only factory designed by architect William Tubby, who's responsible for some of Brooklyn's finest late-19th-century houses. The former firehouse at #225–227, a residence that has kept the red garage door, was built around 1855.

● Proceed across Bridge St. and back into Dumbo. On the right at Jay, Pedro's Spanish American Restaurant features cheap Latin eats and live Cuban music on Sundays. Cross Jay for one of Dumbo's busiest, and hippest, streets. On your left are the luxurious new J condos and adjacent retailers representing the cutting edge in food and art that's a Dumbo specialty: the Spring gallery is both exhibitor and vendor of funky art pieces; Superfine restaurant relies on organic farms and greenmarkets for its fresh, seasonal ingredients. On your right you'll find P.S. Bookshop, a secondhand dealer specializing in first editions and rare volumes, and Retreat, a multifaceted dining destination comprising a coffee bar on the ground floor and a tapas bar upstairs, along with a lounge where even nondiners are welcome.

● You're beneath the bridge again while walking from Pearl to Adams St. On the next block, between two gourmet groceries, are the Loopy Mango clothing and jewelry boutique and the Front Street Galleries. The building at the far corner with Washington was No. 6 of 10 built over a 40-year period by Robert Gair, a Scottish immigrant who was first a successful cardboard box manufacturer and then a commercial real-estate developer. Several of his buildings still have his name and their respective numbers carved in the façades.

● Turn right on Washington St. There's an extraordinary photo op at Water St.: if you wait till there's no traffic (not as difficult here as in most other places in the city) and stand in the middle of the street, the Empire State Building is visible between the columns of the Manhattan Bridge. Gair building No. 1, constructed in the 1880s of brick rather than the reinforced concrete usually used by Gair, is now the Brookwood apartments at 25 Washington St. At the left corner with Plymouth St., you can visit Smack Mellon for unconventional art installations and a good example of warehouse turned gallery space.

*On Washington St. in Dumbo*

- Turn left on Plymouth and behold a superb view of the Brooklyn Bridge. The tracks on the street belonged to a rail system that transported goods between Gair's facilities.

- Turn left on Main St. Bubby's restaurant is popular for weddings, weekend brunch, and, most of all, pies: chocolate peanut butter, sour cherry, and whiskey apple are among the best-sellers. Next to Bubby's is Dumbo's most recognizable landmark, the Clocktower Building. Built in 1914, it was the final (and tallest) Gair building but now bears the name Walentas, the developer who converted all 12 floors, plus the four-story clocktower, into outlandishly priced condos. Diagonally across Water St. is another illustrious Dumbo building turned into condos—the Sweeney Building at 30 Main St., which was a nickelware factory when it opened in 1911. On the left corner of Main and Water, art books are sold and art is exhibited and performed at the powerHouse Arena.

- Turn right on Water to check out two places that helped put Dumbo on the map, Jacques Torres Chocolate and St. Ann's Warehouse, both on your left opposite the Empire Stores building, a former coffee warehouse. At Jacques Torres, you can test your willpower watching bonbons being made, and if you cave, there are as many as 30 kinds of truffles to choose from, plus cookies and everything from corn flakes to candied ginger covered in chocolate. The most famous product, though, is the Wicked Hot Chocolate, infused with cinnamon and a hint of chili pepper. St. Ann's is an avant-garde performance space that relocated from Brooklyn Heights in 2000. Also on this block, you can view but not ride a Roaring '20s carousel that's been restored in the hopes of finding a home in Brooklyn's riverfront park.

- Turn left on Dock St., a short thoroughfare still paved with Belgian blocks.

- Turn left on Front, then right on Washington, passing another former building of the Thomson Meter Company.

- Turn left on York. When you're crossing Pearl, look to your right for the aerial bridges between buildings, which were all part of the Gair complex. Continue on York back to Jay and the subway station where you arrived.

## POINTS OF INTEREST

**Jan Larsen Art** 63 Pearl St., Brooklyn, NY 11201, 718-797-2557

**Halcyon** 57 Pearl St., Brooklyn, NY 11201, 718-260-9299

**Journey** 166 Water St., Brooklyn, NY 11201, 718-797-9277

**Pedro's Spanish American Restaurant** 73 Jay St., Brooklyn, NY 11201, 718-625-0031

**Spring** 126 Front St., Brooklyn, NY 11201, 718-222-1054

**Superfine** 126 Front St., Brooklyn, NY 11201, 718-243-9005

**P.S. Bookshop** 145 Front St., Brooklyn, NY 11201, 718-222-3340

**Retreat** 147 Front St., Brooklyn, NY 11201, 718-797-2322

**Loopy Mango** 117 Front St., Brooklyn, NY 11201, 718-858-5930

**Front Street Galleries** 111 Front St., Brooklyn, NY 11201

**Smack Mellon** 92 Plymouth St., Brooklyn, NY 11201, 718-834-8761

**Bubby's** 1 Main St., Brooklyn, NY 11201, 718-222-0666

**Powerhouse Arena** 37 Main St., Brooklyn, NY 11201, 718-666-3049

**Jacques Torres Chocolate** 66 Water St., Brooklyn, NY 11201, 718-875-9772

**St. Ann's Warehouse** 38 Water St., Brooklyn, NY 11201, 718-858-2424

# route summary

1. Begin at York and Jay Sts. and head west on York.
2. Turn right on Pearl St.
3. Turn right on Water St.
4. Turn right on Bridge St.
5. Turn left on York.
6. Turn left on Navy St., which becomes Hudson Ave.
7. Turn right on Evans St.
8. Turn left on Little St., then left on Plymouth St., and left again on Hudson Ave.
9. Turn right on Water, then left on Gold.
10. Cross Front St., go halfway down the street, then turn around and return to Front and turn left.
11. Turn right on Washington St.
12. Turn left on Plymouth.
13. Turn left on Main St.
14. Turn right on Water.
15. Turn left on Dock St.
16. Turn left on Front, then right on Washington.
17. Turn left on York and return to your starting point.

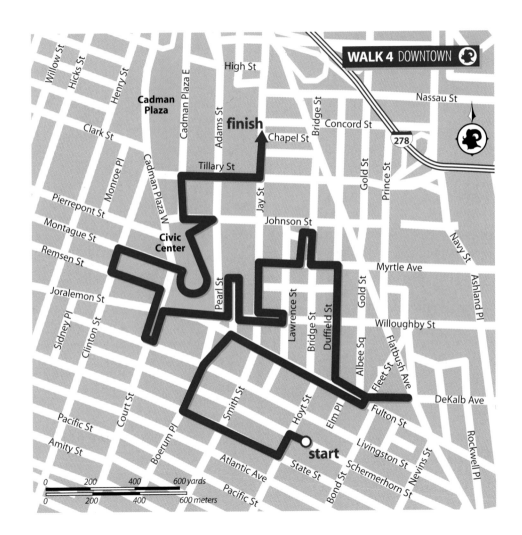

Willow St
Hicks St
Henry St
Cadman Plaza E
High St
Nassau St
Cadman Plaza
Clark St
Adams St
finish
Bridge St
Concord St
Chapel St
Monroe Pl
Cadman Plaza W
Tillary St
Gold St
Prince St
278
Pierrepont St
Jay St
Montague St
Johnson St
Civic Center
Remsen St
Myrtle Ave
Navy St
Joralemon St
Pearl St
Ashland Pl
Sidney Pl
Clinton St
Lawrence St
Bridge St
Duffield St
Gold St
Willoughby St
Court St
Albee Sq
Flatbush Ave
Smith St
Hoyt St
Elm Pl
Fleet St
DeKalb Ave
Pacific St
Boerum Pl
Fulton St
Rockwell Pl
Amity St
Atlantic Ave
State St
Bond St
Schermerhorn St
Livingston St
Nevins St
start
Pacific St

0   200   400   600 yards
0   200   400   600 meters

# 4 DOWNTOWN: CIVIC HUB OF a METROPOLIS

**BOUNDARIES: State St., Clinton St., High St., Flatbush Ave.**
**DISTANCE: Approx. 2½ miles**
**SUBWAY: A or C to Hoyt–Schermerhorn**

Aside from those Brooklynites still squawking about the "mistake of '98," Downtown holds the most reminders that Brooklyn used to be a separate city: government buildings, a concentration of shops and banks, and many former offices of public agencies. After Brooklyn consolidated with Manhattan and three other boroughs to form the City of New York in 1898, Downtown ceased to be the seat of a metropolis and slid into a decades-long decline. But with Brooklyn on the rise again and astronomical rents driving some corporations out of Manhattan, Downtown is reclaiming its stature. The 1990s brought MetroTech, a redeveloped 16-acre corridor encompassing office towers, a new campus for Polytechnic Institute, and public park space, plus the opening of Brooklyn's first hotel (Marriott) since the Depression. In 2003, the city announced plans to develop 4.5 million square feet of office space and create 18,500 jobs in Downtown. Someday soon, Brooklyn's newest and oldest locales may be sitting side-by-side in Downtown.

- From the subway, walk one block south on Hoyt St. and turn right at State St. The State Street Houses comprise 23 Greek Revival and Italianate residences, recognized by both the city landmarks commission and the National Register of Historic Places. Most of them are on your left, #290–#324, but they also include #291–#299 on your right. They were built over a 30-year period (1847–74) and have been meticulously preserved, including the original cast-iron balconies outside #293–#297.

- At Boerum Pl., cross over to the building with the statue out front of children with St. Vincent, the patron saint of charity. A 125-year-old social-services organization named for him is housed inside and was originally an orphanage. Jonathan Lethem's best-selling novel *Motherless Brooklyn,* about four boys who live at St. Vincent's School for Boys, brought the place renewed attention.

- Walk north on Boerum to Schermerhorn St. At the corner on your right, the plain red-brick structure is the Friends Meeting House, used since it was built in 1857 by the Quakers, the religious society committed to peace and justice. Diagonally across Boerum, find the New York Transit Museum—a must for nostalgists, transportation buffs, and museumgoers who like to touch as well as look. The collection includes old buses, turnstiles, trolley models, transit-themed artwork, and vintage subway cars that visitors can board.

● Proceed north to Livingston, then take Red Hook Ln. to your right. This alley, endangered by new construction, predates all development in Brooklyn: it started as a Native American trail and was a strategic route during the American Revolution. It will lead you to the Fulton Street Mall, where you turn right. Go inside T.G.I. Friday's restaurant on your right. The NEW YORK'S OLDEST RESTAURANT etched on the window refers to Gage & Tollner, the building's occupant from 1892 to 2004, who created its sumptuous Victorian ambience, complete with cherrywood-framed mirrors, embossed walls, brass chandeliers, and mahogany tables. Friday's has not, however, retained Gage & Tollner's specialty: clam bellies on toast.

● Continuing along Fulton St., after Smith St. on your right there's a side entrance to the Brooklyn Tabernacle, which fills up its 3,000-seat auditorium for Sunday gospel services. Its 250-person choir won a 1996 Grammy Award. The chain and discount stores of the Fulton mall occupy architecturally distinguished quarters. On your right past Gallatin Pl. is Macy's, formerly Abraham & Straus, or A&S (a retailer that lasted until 1995). Founder Abraham Abraham is credited with inventing the department-store concept, and his store was once the largest in the city. This Art Deco masterpiece, on his store's original site, was designed in 1929 by the architects of Saks Fifth Avenue and Bloomingdale's in Manhattan. Farther down Fulton, note the onion-domed turret and terra cotta urns along the top of the Kay Jewelers building; the metalwork in the balconies, window bays, and finials above Bakers; and the marvelous upper-level ornamentation of Conway's 1890 building.

● Go left onto DeKalb Ave. at the triangle, toward the marble temple erected by the Dime Savings Bank in 1908. Its exterior detail includes an arrangement of Ionic columns, carved bronze doors—the Brooklyn Bridge is one of the images—and a sculpture above the entry of two men along with symbols of agriculture (bearded guy leaning on a bundle of chaffs) and industry (cogs below the clock). The interior is fabulous too: a rotunda of red marble columns with gilded capitals, inlaid with giant dimes, and marble benches engraved with adages about thrift. Follow DeKalb past the bank to the corner of Flatbush Ave. for Junior's, a Brooklyn culinary landmark. The menu is huge and everything is delicious, but it's the cheesecake that justly made this restaurant famous.

- Turn around and walk back on DeKalb and then Fulton. Albee Square, where they meet, was named for the RKO Albee movie palace, built in the 1920s by vaudeville impresario Edward Albee (who also built Broadway's Palace Theatre). Shortly before the cinema was razed in 1977, it screened *Who's Afraid of Virginia Woolf?*, a film based on the play by Albee's namesake grandson.

- Turn right on Duffield St. In 2004 the city notified residents here that their homes would be replaced by commercial development, but the owners of #227 and #233, on your right, say their 150-year-old houses were stops on the Underground Railroad and should be preserved. Across Willoughby St., next to St. Boniface church (1854), are four houses that faced a similar fate in the late 1980s, when MetroTech was planned. These mid-19th-century charmers were saved by being relocated from a few blocks north.

- At Myrtle Ave., the Chase bank on your right is the second-tallest building in Brooklyn, at 450 feet. Go to your left to enter MetroTech. Turn right at Bridge St. The Wunsch Student Center of Polytechnic Institute, on your right, is in an 1846 church that housed Brooklyn's first black congregation (Bridge Street AME, which still exists in Bedford-Stuyvesant) and was a station on the Underground Railroad. Turn around and walk through the MetroTech Commons, a plaza with trees, seating, and public

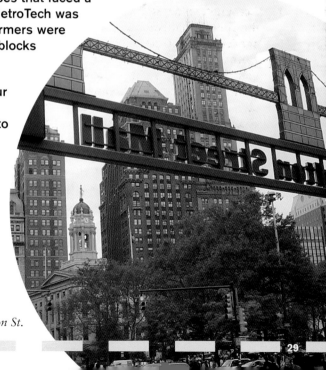

*Approaching the Civic Center from Fulton St.*

art, including some permanent sculptures by Brooklyn-based, Midwestern-born artist Tom Otterness. His piece in front of 2 MetroTech illustrates the local urban legend about alligators in the sewers. Look for another Otterness critter amid the lampposts lining the Commons.

● Proceed west through MetroTech along Myrtle and turn left on Jay St. On your left, sandwiched between mundane contemporary buildings, is a Romanesque Revival composition with two triangular roofs, the higher one atop a story fronted by a receding arch. It was built as headquarters for the Brooklyn fire department in 1892, when firefighters located fires from the tower and then rushed to them via horse-drawn carriage—hence the broad entryway.

● Turn left on Willoughby to see another former headquarters on your left at Lawrence St. The objects depicted in stone around the doorway tell you which agency it served: the telephone company (note the initials carved above the door). Step back to take in the full Beaux Arts splendor of this 1898 structure, then walk back in the direction you came on Willoughby.

● Turn right on Pearl St. In 1867, Quakers started a school in the basement of their meeting house that you saw on Schermerhorn St. In 1973, it moved into Brooklyn Law School's former building on your right. Doorway reliefs depict milestones in world legal history, including the Code of Hammurabi, Ten Commandments, Magna Carta, and U.S. Constitution. The 1929 building is Art Deco with Romanesque influences . . . or vice versa. Pearl dead-ends, so turn around and go back to Willoughby.

● Turn right on Willoughby. Cross Adams St. and walk on Joralemon St., between the Municipal Building and the back of Borough Hall. Turn left on Court St. As on Fulton, the clamor at street level precludes many passersby from looking at the magnificent structures above the shops and eateries. Check out the neo-Gothic skyscraper on your right at the corner of Court and Livingston, then go back toward Joralemon. The Temple Bar Building at 44 Court St. was Brooklyn's tallest when erected in 1901 and is still many people's favorite in the borough, especially because of its cupolas.

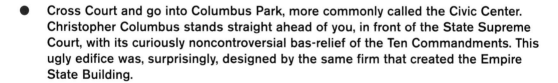

- Turn left on Remsen St. The building at #180 was headquarters of the gas company from 1857 until 1914, when the utility built #176. Both beautiful buildings are now used by St. Francis College.

- Turn right on Clinton St. The next street, Montague, has been Bank Row since the 19th century, though the banks all have new names. Chase occupies a 1915 building that was modeled on a palace in Verona, Italy, and features extraordinary ornamentation on its wrought-iron gates, entryway, and lampposts, as well as a gilded ceiling inside. Citibank has the 1903 beaut next to it, which was designed by the same architects as the Dime you saw near Fulton. The Art Deco skyscraper at #185 was designed by architects who would next work on Rockefeller Center.

- Cross Court and go into Columbus Park, more commonly called the Civic Center. Christopher Columbus stands straight ahead of you, in front of the State Supreme Court, with its curiously noncontroversial bas-relief of the Ten Commandments. This ugly edifice was, surprisingly, designed by the same firm that created the Empire State Building.

- Go to your right toward Borough Hall. This exquisite Greek Revival structure opened in 1849 as Brooklyn's City Hall. It lost its original cupola to a fire in 1895, and the replacement went up in 1898, with a flag on top. Lady Justice was just added in 1987.

- With your back to Borough Hall, walk the length of the plaza, which is as close a facsimile of a European piazza as you're likely to find in NYC. Between the fountain and the Columbus statue, you'll find a bust of Robert F. Kennedy, once the state's U.S. senator; a tree planted in memory of President John F. Kennedy; and a monument to Washington Roebling, engineer of the Brooklyn Bridge. The sculptor of the RFK bust also created the plaque commemorating philanthropist Cornelius Heeney that's on your left after you pass the subway kiosks. You can see the Manhattan Bridge off in the distance as you approach the north end of the Civic Center, which features a statue of Henry Ward Beecher, abolitionist pastor of nearby Church of the Pilgrims. Beyond the Beecher statue, the Romanesque fortress with a pot-bellied arcade at the top of the tower was built by the U.S. Postal Service in 1891. Walk on Johnson St. to see its turrets, then go north past the front of it on Cadman Plaza E.

- Turn right on Tillary St., then go left on Jay and proceed to Chapel St. The walk ends where worship began for Long Island's Roman Catholics. Before St. James was established in 1822, Catholics who lived in Brooklyn and the rest of Long Island had to travel to Manhattan for services.

- Across the street from the church, take the B67 or B75 bus back to the Jay St.– Borough Hall subway station at the Fulton Mall.

## POINTS OF INTEREST

**New York Transit Museum** Boerum Pl. and Schermerhorn St., Brooklyn, NY 11201, 718-694-1600

**Dime Savings Bank (Washington Mutual)** 9 DeKalb Ave., Brooklyn, NY 11201, 718-403-7900

**Junior's** Flatbush and DeKalb Aves., Brooklyn, NY 11201, 718-852-5257

# route summary

1. Walk south on Hoyt St. from the subway and turn right on State St.
2. Turn right on Boerum Pl.
3. Go to the right on Red Hook Ln. from Boerum and Livingston St.
4. Go right on Fulton St., then onto DeKalb Ave.; backtrack via DeKalb from Junior's.
5. From Fulton turn right on Duffield St.
6. Make a left on Myrtle St. into MetroTech.
7. Turn right on Bridge St., then walk through the Commons back to Myrtle and go west.
8. Turn left on Jay St.
9. Go left on Willoughby St. to Lawrence St., then turn around.
10. Turn right on Pearl St., walk to its end, then turn around.
11. Turn right Willoughby, which becomes Joralemon St.
12. Turn left on Court St.; then at Livingston turn around and walk north.
13. Turn left on Remsen St.
14. Turn right on Clinton St., then right on Montague St.
15. Cross Court St. into Columbus Park.
16. Walk around the plaza, exiting north onto Cadman Plaza E.
17. Turn right on Tillary St.
18. Go left on Jay to Chapel St.
19. Take the bus south on Jay for the A, C, or F train at Jay St.–Borough Hall.

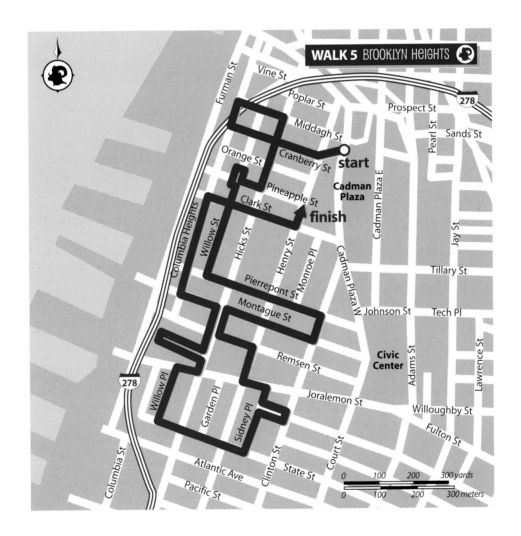

**WALK 5 Brooklyn Heights**

Furman St
Vine St
Poplar St
Middagh St
Cranberry St
Orange St
Pineapple St
Clark St
Columbia Heights
Willow St
Hicks St
Henry St
Monroe Pl
Pierrepont St
Montague St
Remsen St
Joralemon St
Willow Pl
Garden Pl
Sidney Pl
Clinton St
State St
Court St
Atlantic Ave
Pacific St
Columbia St
278
278
Prospect St
Pearl St
Sands St
Cadman Plaza E
Cadman Plaza W
Tillary St
Johnson St
Tech Pl
Civic Center
Adams St
Willoughby St
Fulton St
Lawrence St
Jay St

**start**
**Cadman Plaza**
**finish**

| 0 | 100 | 200 | 300 yards |
| 0 | 100 | 200 | 300 meters |

# 5 Brooklyn Heights: Epitome of 19th-Century Gentility

BOUNDARIES: **Middagh St., Columbia Heights, State St., Clinton St.**
DISTANCE: **Approx. 3 miles**
SUBWAY: **A or C to High St.**

Brooklyn Heights needs no introduction, since it's the one place in Brooklyn likely to have been visited by tourists and residents of the other boroughs. It's even recognizable to those who haven't been here, through its numerous appearances in movies, from *Moonstruck* to *Prizzi's Honor* to *The Verdict* (where it stood in for Boston). It also needs no introduction in the sense that its gloriousness speaks for itself. There are more than 600 antebellum homes in the neighborhood, a slew of spectacular churches, and small streets that ooze charm. In 1965 the entire neighborhood gained landmark status—the first historic district recognized by the city—and that designation curtailed any new construction out of scale with the existing buildings. The Heights was the first American suburb, made feasible when Robert Fulton launched his ferry from Manhattan in 1814. Then, as now, it was a place of affluence.

● Exit the subway on **Cadman Plaza W.** The plaza in front of the apartments here was the approximate location of the Rome brothers' print shop, where Walt Whitman set type in 1855 for his first edition of *Leaves of Grass*.

● Walk between the apartments to **Henry St.**, then continue west on **Cranberry St.** On the right are Greek Revival brickfronts at #65–#67 and #45–#53. In between them is the Church of the Assumption, established in 1842. The parish lost its original building, located farther east, when the Manhattan Bridge was constructed and erected this neo-Renaissance church in 1908. After crossing Willow St., the star of an Oscar-winning movie is on your right. The corner house, #19, was used for exterior shots of Cher's home in *Moonstruck.* Cranberry is the street where Cher kicked a can as she dreamily strolled home after her night at the opera.

● Turn right at the **Fruit Street Sitting Area.** The historic marker tells of the century-spanning effort to introduce a promenade into Brooklyn Heights (and also explains the fruit nomenclature of nearby streets). Though the Promenade that begins just a block over is the Heights' showpiece, the people who live on this stretch of Columbia Heights practically have their own private esplanade with this little park, since it gets few visitors but offers the same incredible vistas.

- Go right on Middagh St., walking around or through Harry Chapin Playground. Singer/humanitarian Chapin, who grew up in the Heights, had his biggest hit with "Cat's in the Cradle." Another popular story-song of his, "Taxi," is represented in the benches. Across Willow on your right, #24 is the oldest house in Brooklyn Heights, constructed in 1824 of wood. Connoisseurs and casual observers alike adore its quarter-round windows on Willow and its Federal-style entryway. Virtually this entire block is composed of early-19th-century wood houses.

- Turn right on Hicks St. There's a story people like to tell: the word "hick" was coined because Manhattan snobs regarded those from across the river, including a family named Hicks, as bumpkins. The story doesn't sound too believable, however, if you consider that the Hicks brothers ran an East River ferry monopoly and owned enough land that they could name a street after themselves. That kind of influence would impress even Manhattanites.

- Turn right on Pineapple St. At Willow, go to the right to see #70, where Truman Capote lived in the basement while he was writing *Breakfast at Tiffany's.* The house, dating to the 1830s, is one of the largest Greek Revival homes in New York and was restored by longtime owner Oliver Smith, the late Broadway set designer who won multiple Tonys (for *West Side Story, My Fair Lady,* and seven other shows).

- Turn around and head south on Willow. After Pineapple, the whole block on your left is consumed by an exquisite building that used to be Brooklyn's priciest hotel, the Leverich Towers, which charged $3 a night in 1931. It's one of several historic buildings in the Heights and Dumbo that have been converted to residence halls for the Jehovah's Witnesses, which is headquartered in the area. The next block of Willow presents a long and lovely assortment of decorating schemes and eras, including Federal, Queen Anne, neo-Gothic, and Tudor stylings. One brownstone on your right houses Dansk Sømandskirke (Danish Seaman's Church), the only church in North America that holds weekly services in Danish. The former carriage house at #151 is said to have been part of the Underground Railroad; that's a redwood tree in its yard.

The Federal classics at #155–#159 were built in the 1820s, before the current street pattern, which is why they don't align with Willow as the other houses do. Playwright Arthur Miller wrote *The Crucible* while living at #155.

● Turn left on Pierrepont St., another outstanding residential street. The most magnificent mansion is on your right at Henry. This Romanesque treasure, marred only by a canopy added in the mid-20th century, was completed in 1890 for manufacturing tycoon Herman Behr (whose son Karl, an attorney and tennis champion, would survive the *Titanic*). It later became a brothel, then a Franciscan monastery and, since the 1970s, a condominium. The Unitarian Church on your left at Pierrepont and Monroe Sts. is the oldest church building in Brooklyn. Its construction in 1844 has been credited with launching the Gothic Revival movement in the United States. The church installed eight Tiffany stained-glass windows for its golden anniversary and the rose window for its centennial. On your right at Clinton St., visit the Brooklyn Historical Society, which mounts exhibitions and owns an invaluable archive and library of books, maps, correspondence, newspapers, census and landholding records, and other Brooklyn artifacts. Across from the historical society, St. Ann's, a progressive private school, occupies a former clubhouse for well-heeled gentlemen, the prestigious Crescent Athletic Club.

● Turn right on Clinton, then right on Montague St., walking around St. Ann and the Holy Trinity. The church's 60 stained-glass windows are considered the country's best and were the first such windows made in America (all by one artist). From this Gothic Revival masterpiece, proceed to the Queen Anne gems of Montague St., on your right past Henry: the adjoining Grosvenor and Berkeley, followed a couple of doors

*Willow St.*

down by the Montague. All three buildings were designed in 1885 by the Parfitt Brothers, who were responsible for many fine churches and homes in late-19th-century Brooklyn. Bob Dylan sang about Montague St. during its scruffier 20th-century phase in "Tangled Up in Blue." Now the street is a gentrified retail district. The gourmet deli Lassen & Hennigs, at #114, names its sandwiches after Brooklyn neighborhoods and also makes soups, salads, and desserts. The kitchenware outlet Fishs Eddy, at #122, sells Brooklynese items—a mug that says *cawffee,* a bowl for *shuguh*—and plates with Brooklyn landmarks on them. On your left before you cross Hicks, Jehovah's Witnesses live in the Bossert, once a hotel lauded as "the Waldorf-Astoria of Brooklyn."

● Go left on Hicks and left again on Remsen St. to Henry. You don't need to be close to Our Lady of Lebanon Maronite Catholic Cathedral, with its Rapunzel's tower, to spot it, but you do want to go up to the entrances on both Remsen and Henry to see its engraved bronze doors. They were salvaged from the *Normandie,* the largest ocean liner in the world, which was being refitted for military deployment during World War II when it caught fire at the dock in Manhattan and capsized. The church's Romanesque style was uncharacteristic for its architect, the Gothic master Richard Upjohn, and was a first for churches in the United States.

● Facing the church, go to your right on Henry. Look down Hunts Ln. to your left, a mews of former carriage houses. The mansion at #236 is a standout on your right.

● Turn left on Joralemon St. Two houses on your left are very different, but both beautiful. First is the limestone-and-brick #129, with broad features and embossment and balustrade ornamentation. The garlands on this 1890 mansion were a popular Victorian flourish. Its plainer, more traditional neighbor on the other side of the apartment building is an exemplar of its own era, the 1830s, when this and several other Federal-style houses were built on this street. It alone survives.

● Turn right on Sidney Pl., named for a 16th-century British statesman and author who never set foot in Brooklyn but had influential admirers here. St. Charles Borromeo, the church on your left with a tall verdigris spire, was erected in 1868. Its architect, Patrick Keely, designed more of America's Catholic churches than anyone else.

- Go left on Aitken Pl. to the next intersection, where Livingston St. takes over for Aitken, to see the dazzling Victorian Gothic church (now a private school) across Clinton. It was designed in the late 1860s by James Renwick Jr. after he had drafted the plans for St. Patrick's Cathedral on 5th Ave. in Manhattan.

- Go back on Aitken to Sidney and turn left, then make a right on State St. Turn right on Willow Pl. Immediately on your right is a group of red-brick townhouses in a so-called colonnade row. An identical quartet was built directly across the street (both in the 1840s), but only one from that row survives. Farther down on the left, the Heights Players, a community theater that's been around for more than 50 years, and the St. Ann's preschool are the tenants of the Unitarian Church's former chapel. Alfred Treadway White, a businessman/heir whose "model tenements" elevated the quality of housing that the working class could afford (one of his projects, Riverside, is on an adjacent street, Columbia Pl.), was the patron of this chapel. It had to be sold upon his death in 1921 and subsequently housed a brothel frequented by Navy Yard employees, then a furniture maker, then a foundry before being rescued by a citizens' rehabilitation campaign in the 1960s.

- Turn right on Joralemon. The 1847 house on your right at #58 has blackened windows because there's nothing in the house except a ventilation shaft for the subway. Don't these upscale neighborhoods always have their secrets behind closed doors?

- Turn left on Hicks. Grace Church on the left proffers another bold design by Richard Upjohn, this one in his more typical Gothic Revival vernacular.

- Turn left on Grace Ct. If you ever needed proof that life isn't fair, here it is. In a city where having any green space to yourself is an impossible dream for millions of people, certain homeowners on Remsen St. have these double-deep back lawns. In a city where one almost always has to sacrifice convenience for peace and quiet, this tranquil, secluded street is just a couple of blocks from a commercial center. And in a city where it can be difficult to afford a home with *any* character at all, these houses have oodles of it. Don't forget the fantastic view of Manhattan and the Statue of Liberty from just outside their doors either! (Go all the way to the end to see it.) There's also a celebrity connection: Arthur Miller wrote *Death of a Salesman* at #31 and later sold the house to civil rights leader W.E.B. DuBois.

- Resume walking north on Hicks, taking note of Grace Ct. Alley to your right, another mews of former carriage houses, these built for the mansions of Joralemon and Remsen Sts.

- Turn left on Montague. The long building on your right with a stepped gable is the Heights Casino. When it was built in 1904, the word "casino" was used for places of various social amusements, not just gambling. This casino was, and is, a renowned racquet club, hosting squash tournaments, producing many squash champions, and containing the first indoor tennis courts in the United States. There's a beautiful apartment building across from it, as well as one at the left corner with Pierrepont Pl. The Romanesque #62 was designed by Montrose Morris, architect of several landmark residences (mostly in Bedford-Stuyvesant).

- Turn right at Pierrepont Pl. The huge Italianate brownstone manses on your left date to 1857. The home at #3 was built for A.A. Low, an übersuccessful importer of tea and silk from Asia, whose son Seth grew up to be the only person ever to serve as mayor of both Brooklyn and New York City. Across Pierrepont St., Pierrepont Pl. becomes Columbia Heights. This enchanting street, whose west side backs up to the Promenade, features one elegant house after another.

- Turn right at Clark St. The subway entrance on Henry is inside the St. George, a hotel that operated from 1929 into the 1960s on a scale with today's Las Vegas megaresorts. Its 2,632 guest rooms were the most of any hotel in the world, and its ballroom, saltwater pool, and rooftop restaurant were legendary. A 1930s guidebook described it as "a good-sized city in itself" and "the social mecca of all Brooklyn." The St. George deteriorated with the rest of Brooklyn in the 1960s and '70s, but has since been rehabilitated and now contains a college dormitory and co-op apartments.

## POINTS OF INTEREST

**Harry Chapin Playground** Columbia Heights and Middagh St., Brooklyn, NY 11201
**Brooklyn Historical Society** 128 Pierrepont St., Brooklyn, NY 11201, 718-222-4111
**Lassen & Hennigs** 114 Montague St., Brooklyn, NY 11201, 718-875-6272

**Fishs Eddy** 122 Montague St., Brooklyn, NY 11201, 718-797-3990

**Heights Players** 26 Willow Pl., Brooklyn, NY 11201, 718-237-2752

## route summary

1. Begin at Cadman Plaza W. and walk west onto Cranberry St.
2. From Cranberry, turn right at Columbia Heights.
3. Go right on Middagh St.
4. Turn right at Hicks St.
5. Turn right on Pineapple St.
6. Turn right on Willow St., then turn around and walk south.
7. Go left on Pierrepont St.
8. Turn right on Clinton St.
9. Turn right on Montague St.
10. Turn left on Hicks.
11. Go left on Remsen St.
12. Turn right at Henry St.
13. Turn left on Joralemon St.
14. Turn right on Sidney Pl.
15. Go left on Aitken Pl. to Clinton St., then go back to Sidney and turn left.
16. Turn right on State St.
17. Turn right on Willow Pl.
18. Turn right on Joralemon.
19. Go left on Hicks.
20. Go left down Grace Ct., then return to Hicks and resume walking north.
21. Turn left on Montague.
22. Turn right on Pierrepont Pl., which leads onto Columbia Heights.
23. Turn right at Clark St. and get the subway at Henry.

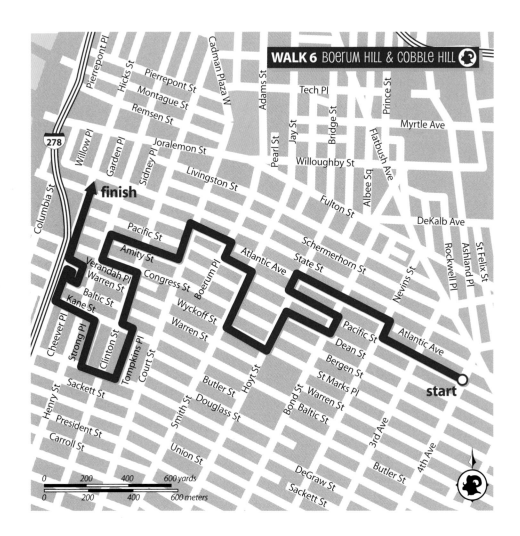

WALK 6 BOERUM HILL & COBBLE HILL

finish

start

Pierrepont Pl
Hicks St
Pierrepont St
Montague St
Remsen St
Cadman Plaza W
Adams St
Tech Pl
Prince St
Myrtle Ave
Jay St
Bridge St
Pearl St
Willoughby St
Flatbush Ave
278
Willow Pl
Garden Pl
Sidney Pl
Joralemon St
Livingston St
Columbia St
Fulton St
Albee Sq
DeKalb Ave
Rockwell Pl
Ashland Pl
St Felix St
Pacific St
Amity St
Verandah Pl
Warren St
Congress St
Boerum Pl
Atlantic Ave
Schermerhorn St
State St
Nevins St
Baltic St
Kane St
Wyckoff St
Warren St
Pacific St
Atlantic Ave
Cheever Pl
Strong Pl
Clinton St
Tompkins Pl
Court St
Hoyt St
Dean St
Bergen St
St Marks Pl
Warren St
Baltic St
Bond St
3rd Ave
4th Ave
Henry St
Sackett St
Butler St
Douglass St
Smith St
Union St
DeGraw St
Sackett St
Butler St
President St
Carroll St

0    200    400    600 yards
0    200    400    600 meters

# 6 BOERUM HILL AND COBBLE HILL: PASSING THE TEST OF TIME

**BOUNDARIES:** **Atlantic Ave., 4th Ave., DeGraw St., Hicks St.**
**DISTANCE:** **Approx. 2 ¾ miles**
**SUBWAY:** **B, D, N, Q, R, 2, 3, or 4 to Atlantic Ave./Pacific St.**

Begin near a large mall of today's most recognizable chain stores. Cross the street and you are transported into the 19th century. Boerum Hill and Cobble Hill, adjacent neighborhoods south of Atlantic Ave., were fashionable districts in the 1870s. The emergence of Smith and Court Sts.—and the rebirth of Atlantic Ave.—as trendy shopping and dining destinations have added a new facet to this area rich in historic homes and churches along tree-lined streets. In recent years Boerum Hill and Cobble Hill have been appended to Carroll Gardens (their neighbor to the south) by acronym-favoring real-estate interests as BoCoCa.

● Exit the subway at Pacific St. and 4th Ave. Bound to catch your eye is the 1870 stone Church of the Redeemer across 4th Ave.

● Go over to the church and walk beside its nave on Pacific St. After some classic brownstones, you'll find on your left the Brooklyn High School of the Arts. The magnet school for math and science next to it, with a marbleized exterior, was formerly a printing plant for *The New York Times.*

● Cross 3rd Ave., where the tannish Bethlehem Lutheran Church has stood since 1894. Next to the church, go into the playground on your left to see a 9/11 memorial painted by local teens on the low wall parallel to Pacific St. After leaving this playground, cross the street to visit the leafier, more intimate North Pacific Playground, which encompasses a community garden.

● Turn right at Nevins St., then left on Atlantic Ave., which slices east-west across the entire borough. This section of it has long been known for Middle Eastern restaurants and antiques shops, and its new look also includes diversified cuisine and hip boutiques. Old-fashioned ambience is preserved in the Victorian storefronts on your left.

On your right, the "Ex-Lax" apartment building, with the sky-blue entranceway, was one of the earliest industrial-to-residential conversions (circa 1980). You'll also pass the Pentecostal House of the Lord, whose pastor, Herbert Daughtry, is a prominent civil rights activist in the city.

● Cross Bond St. and you're in the midst of antiques dealers. Speaking of old things: look for floral, shell, and rope designs in doorways, window frames, and cornices—all typical of the Victorian era when the street developed commercially. Indulge your sweet tooth at Downtown Atlantic on the left, with its scrumptious assortment of cupcakes and tarts.

● Turn left on Hoyt St., but not before at least peeking into Hoyt Street Garden at the corner. This oasis was created in 1975, when the area was in shabby condition. The land's owner, the Presbyterian church beside it on Atlantic Ave., has given community volunteers complete control over the garden for free. This arrangement may not last— the Spanish-speaking congregation is hard up for funds, having dwindled significantly as gentrification has driven out many parishioners, and it may sell the space.

● Turn left at Pacific and go into the Bishop Francis J. Mugavero Center for Geriatric Care on the right. The history here is in the lobby, where two display cases contain antique household items unearthed when the nursing home was built in the early 1990s. Continuing east on Pacific, you'll see yellow-brick Cuyler Church, built in the 1890s and now residential. Next to the ex-church, the white house (with colonnaded porch) dared to be different from the brick and brownstone houses (with stoops) surrounding it, though they all date to the same period. The house at #347 also broke with the prevalent Greek and Renaissance Revival styles—and got its bronze balcony off another house.

● Turn right at Bond and proceed to Dean St., smack in the middle of Boerum Hill's historic district. In both directions Dean is a tranquil tree-lined street of genteel 19th-century rowhouses; go to the right. Poet Sidney Lanier, who's strongly identified with the South, lived at #195 in late 1874 and from this brownstone rhapsodized about Georgia farmland in his poem "Corn."

- Turn left at Hoyt. The Brooklyn Inn on the southwest corner at Bergen St. was a speakeasy during Prohibition. The interior of the bar features woodwork and stained glass that were shipped from Europe. The building itself dates to about 1850, its exterior ironwork to the 1880s.

- Turn right on Wyckoff St. The artistic bent of Boerum Hill is represented by the house at #108, whose façade, stoop, pavement, even window bars are covered with a mosaic of tiles, beads, mirrors, and shells.

- Turn right on Smith St., the ballyhooed restaurant row of Brooklyn. In just the three blocks to Pacific, you get a good idea of the dining variety available. For a quick boost, have them whip up a health drink for you at Cafe Kai, on your right between Wyckoff and Bergen. There are also a lot of specialty shops—and a kicky museum on your right between Dean and Pacific. The Micro Museum specializes in interactive art, often involving audiovisual components and furniture.

- Turn left on Pacific, then right on Boerum Pl. When you're back at Atlantic Ave., turn left. You're walking on top of something listed on the National Register of Historic Places: a rail tunnel, extending a ½ mile to the waterfront, that was constructed in 1844. It was largely forgotten—except, allegedly, by bootleggers and other underworld personages—until a local train buff had it excavated around 1980. Going back farther in time, the bank at the corner of Atlantic and Court was the site of a fort whose role in the American Revolution is commemorated in a plaque on Court.

- Turn left on Court. BookCourt, on your left past Pacific, is a general bookstore that stocks a lot of

*Hoyt Street Garden*

Brooklyn-related titles. Turn right on Amity St. and you're in the Cobble Hill historic district. Miss Jeanette Jerome (later known as Jennie Churchill, the American socialite mother of Winston) was born at 197 Amity St. But the house on the left at Amity and Clinton Sts. is the jewel in Cobble Hill's crown: the DeGraw mansion, with its large backyard, was built in 1845 and once had a view of the water. Approaching Henry St. on Amity, the busily embellished Dudley Memorial opened as a nurses' dormitory in 1902 and now is part of Long Island College Hospital, as is the former Polhemus Dispensary across Henry. Its Latin inscription translates to "Knowledge is the friend of the poor."

● Turn left on Henry. Across Congress St., the entire west side of the block is occupied by another architecturally eminent medical facility—Cobble Hill Health Center, now a nursing home but built as a church-affiliated charity hospital in 1888.

● Turn left on Verandah Pl. Charming Cobble Hill Park is on your left, across from a row of 1850s homes, including the one at #40 that Thomas Wolfe, who lived there in 1930, described in *You Can't Go Home Again.*

● Go right on Clinton. The 1843 house with slightly thrust windows at #296, on your right as you near Baltic St., was designed by Richard Upjohn, a leading architect of the Gothic Revival movement, who lived here while his most famous project, Manhattan's Trinity Church, was being built. Upjohn was also architect of Christ Church, one block farther at Clinton and Kane Sts. This 1842 masterpiece, with a 120-foot, four-spire steeple, is the oldest Episcopal church building in Brooklyn, and its altar, pulpit, and some windows were designed by Tiffany.

● Turn left at Kane and proceed to another longstanding house of worship. The Kane Street Synagogue, home to Brooklyn's oldest Jewish congregation, was built in 1856 as a Dutch Reformed church.

● Turn right on Tompkins Pl. and right on DeGraw St. Then turn right and walk down lovely Strong Pl. to Kane and turn left. Go to your right at Hicks St. You'll pass the Home apartments between Kane and Baltic Sts., then the Tower building on the other side of Baltic. These "model tenements" went up in the late 1870s, providing those of modest means with decent plumbing and ventilation for the first time.

● Turn right on Warren St. to see another landmark in working-class housing. Warren Pl., a mews on your right, was developed in 1878–79 by the same businessman responsible for the Tower and Home buildings—he'd been enlightened about London's experiments in upgraded worker housing by the newspaper reports of local journalist Walt Whitman. These former "Cottages for Workingmen" are today affordable only to those with incomes far above workingmen's. Take one path through Warren Pl. when you enter and the other on your way out.

● Turn left on Warren St. and head back to Hicks, taking note of the stained-glass windows in the brick church on your right. Turn right on Hicks and you'll see that the entire church looks fabulous for an antebellum construction . . . probably because the 1860 building has been refurbished and converted into apartments. Proceed on Hicks to Upper Van Voorhees Park, on your left at Amity. Slivered between a parking garage, highway, and hospital, this verdant park proves that any patch of urban acreage can be beautified.

● Exit the park at its north end and turn left. Back on Atlantic Ave., board the B63 bus to return to your starting point and transfer to the subway.

## POINTS OF INTEREST

**Downtown Atlantic** 364 Atlantic Ave., Brooklyn, NY 11217, 718-852-9945

**North Pacific Playground** Pacific St. between 3rd Ave. and Nevins St., Brooklyn, NY 11217

**Hoyt Street Garden** Hoyt St. at Atlantic Ave., Brooklyn, NY 11217

**Brooklyn Inn** 138 Bergen St., Brooklyn, NY 11217, 718-625-9741

**Cafe Kai** 151 Smith St., Brooklyn, NY 11201, 718-596-3466

**Micro Museum** 123 Smith St., Brooklyn, NY 11201, 718-797-3116

**South Brooklyn Savings Institution (Sovereign Bank)** 130 Court St. at Atlantic Ave., Brooklyn, NY 11201

**BookCourt** 163 Court St., Brooklyn, NY 11201, 718-875-3677

**Cobble Hill Park** Clinton St. and Verandah Pl., Brooklyn, NY 11201

**Upper Van Voorhees Park** Hicks St. between Atlantic Ave. and Congress St., Brooklyn, NY 11201

## route summary

1.   Begin at 4th Ave. and Pacific St. and walk west on Pacific.
2.   Turn right on Nevins St., then left on Atlantic Ave.
3.   Turn left on Hoyt St.
4.   Turn left on Pacific.
5.   Turn right on Bond St., then right on Dean St.
6.   Turn left on Hoyt.
7.   Turn right on Wyckoff St.
8.   Turn right on Smith St.
9.   Turn left on Pacific, right on Boerum Pl., and then left on Atlantic.
10.  Turn left on Court St., then right on Amity St.
11.  Turn left on Henry St.
12.  Turn left on Verandah Pl.
13.  Turn right on Clinton St.
14.  Turn left on Kane St.
15.  Turn right on Tompkins Pl. and right on DeGraw St. Turn right on Strong Pl. to Kane and go left, then turn right on Hicks.
16.  Turn right on Warren St. Go in and out of Warren Pl. to your right, then left on Warren St.
17.  Go right on Hicks to Atlantic and catch the B63 bus back to the subway.

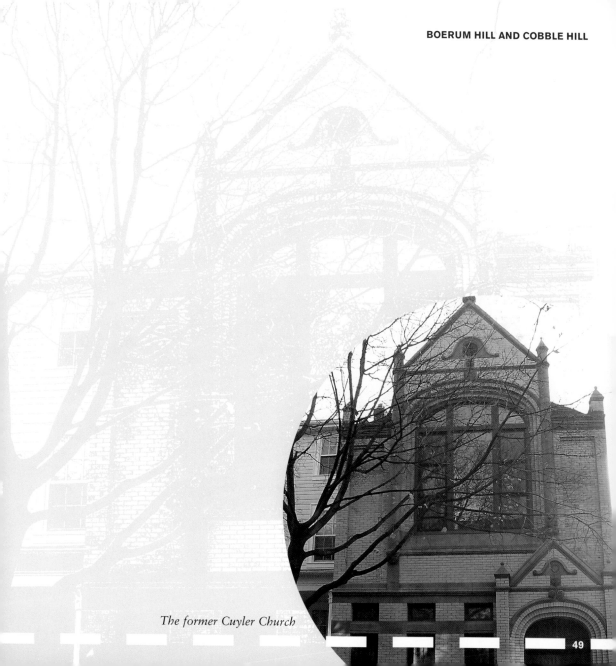

*The former Cuyler Church*

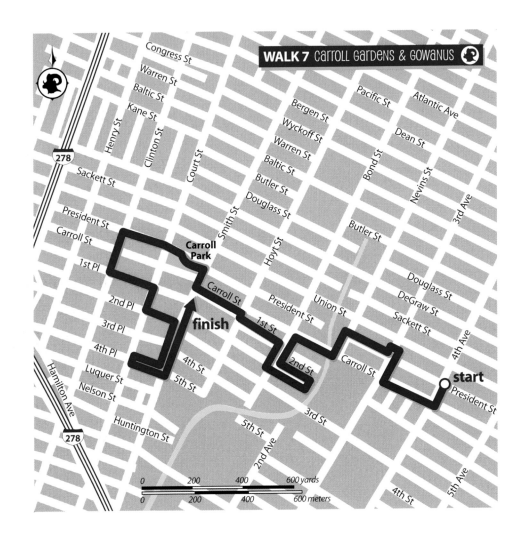

WALK 7 CARROLL GARDENS & GOWANUS

Congress St
Warren St
Baltic St
Kane St
Henry St
Clinton St
Court St
Sackett St
President St
Carroll St
1st Pl
2nd Pl
3rd Pl
4th Pl
Luquer St
Nelson St
Huntington St
Hamilton Ave
278
278

Bergen St
Wyckoff St
Warren St
Baltic St
Butler St
Douglass St
Smith St
Hoyt St
Carroll St
President St
1st St
2nd St
4th St
5th St
3rd St
5th St
2nd Ave
4th St

Pacific St
Atlantic Ave
Dean St
Bond St
Nevins St
3rd Ave
Butler St
Douglass St
DeGraw St
Union St
Sackett St
Carroll St
4th Ave
5th Ave

Carroll
Park

finish

start
President St

0      200      400      600 yards
0      200      400      600 meters

# 7  Carroll Gardens and Gowanus: a Man, a Plan, a Canal

**BOUNDARIES: 4th Ave., Union St., Clinton St., 4th Pl.**
**DISTANCE: Approx. 2 miles**
**SUBWAY: R to Union St.**

The "Carroll" comes from Declaration of Independence signatory Charles Carroll; the "Gardens" from the neighborhood design conceived by surveyor Richard Butts in 1846. The houses' deep front yards have been well cared for over the years by garden-loving Italians, who moved here for the longshore work and were the dominant immigrant group throughout the 20th century. With its proximity to Manhattan and abundance of brownstones, Carroll Gardens more recently has been a magnet for yuppies—who transformed once-mundane Smith St. into a vaunted destination for boutique shopping and haute cuisine. Yet the Italian imprint has not eroded completely in either Carroll Gardens or Gowanus, the grittier 'hood across the canal. Long ignored because of its association with the festering canal, Gowanus is yet another Brooklyn neighborhood that's being rediscovered by artists staking out non-Manhattan turf.

● Exit the subway on Gowanus's border with Park Slope, 4th Ave. To the north: a full-length view of the Williamsburgh Savings Bank tower in Fort Greene. Close-by to the south: the Brooklyn Lyceum, an arts center (the Brooklyn Underground Film Festival is one of its programs) that's taken up residence in the former Public Bath No. 7, which was built circa 1907 and boasts a sea-themed façade. Walk south.

● Turn right on Carroll St. On your left, drop into a simple community garden named for Gil Hodges, the beloved Dodger first baseman. Across Denton Pl. is Our Lady of Peace Roman Catholic Church, where a young Frank Sinatra supposedly sang at a charity event in the 1940s. As you cross Whitwell Pl., look to your left to see a commercial relic: the Eagle Clothes sign (you'll see it from the back). Once upon a time, these neon-on-metal advertisements peppered the area.

● Turn right on 3rd Ave. Glory Social Club on your left is the only survivor of its kind. The neighborhood used to be full of such "no girls allowed" hangouts for *paisans*.

Membership dues are just $5 a month at Glory, which has been around since 1927. Across President St., Canal Bar may seem of a similar vintage, but it just opened in 2005. The young owners installed an 80-year-old mahogany bar and assorted maritime objects to capture the ambience of a waterfront dive. They barbecue out front every Sunday afternoon—even in snowstorms—and the grub is free to drinkers.

● Go back the few steps to President and head west. As you near Nevins St., you may start smelling wax; the Crusader Candle Co. keeps its doors open in warmer weather, and you may get a look inside at the assembly line after turning left on Nevins.

● Go right on Carroll St. Cross the Gowanus Canal on the wood planks of the oldest (1889) of four retractile bridges left in the country. These days the canal is placid and more or less tolerable fragrance-wise, thanks to an expensive and ambitious cleanup effort. In the 1840s a natural creek was extended by a mile or so to create the canal for mercantile access to the bay. A residential neighborhood developed around the canal, which cargo transporters relied on for about a century until the Gowanus Expressway rendered it obsolete. Unused for the second half of the 20th century, the canal putrefied, but it now has a sewage-treatment plant and is flushed regularly with clean water. Across the bridge, the old industrial silo on your left has been converted into the Issue Project Room, a venue for music performances, poetry readings, and other eclectic arts events.

● Turn left on Bond St. and left on 2nd St. to reach the Gowanus Dredgers operation. This environmental group offers canoes and kayaks for free public use on weekends. Thanks to the initiative of folks like the Dredgers, people have started envisioning a recreational and retail esplanade along the canal.

● Go back to Bond and turn right. Turn left on 1st St. As you walk uphill, shabbier conditions give way to pleasant residential surroundings. When you reach Hoyt St., you're within Carroll Gardens' historic district, developed entirely between 1869 and 1884.

● Turn right on Hoyt, then left on Carroll. Turn right on Smith St., but not before looking in the corner storefront on your right. This window plus two more on Smith comprise gallerythe.org, which eschews indoor space in favor of purveying art to all passersby.

- Proceed on Smith to President and enter Carroll Park to your left. A private garden in Richard Butts's plan for the neighborhood, Carroll Park was developed as a city park in 1867. Go to your right as you enter and note the distances to poles and oceans marked on the ground. Walk between playgrounds to the World War I memorial. The Italian influence is evident in the bocce alley alongside the basketball courts in front of you.

- Leave the park via the path to your right from the war monument. Turn left onto President, with its lovely brownstones and the former South Congregational church at the far corner with Court St. Stay on President, but glimpse the neighborhood in transition to your right at Court: on one side, an Internet cafe, health-food store, and gym serve the yuppie influx; across from them, a fish market, G. Esposito butcher/deli (in operation since 1922), Fratelli Ravioli, and Marco Polo restaurant preserve the Italian flavor. West of the ex-church on President, the congregation now worships in the building at #257, originally constructed (in 1889) as the ladies parlor. Next to it, the magnificent 1893 home at #255—five stories of stone and curved brick—used to be the rectory.

- Turn left on Clinton. St. Paul's Episcopal sits on your left at Carroll St. On your right, the F.G. Guido Funeral Home is considered the finest example of Greek Revival architecture in all of New York City. The house was built for John Rankin in 1840.

- Turn left on 1st Pl., one of the streets in Richard Butts's initial plan (which covered 1st through 4th Pl. but was extended to President St.).

- Turn right on Court, then left on 2nd Pl., another street with large garden yards.

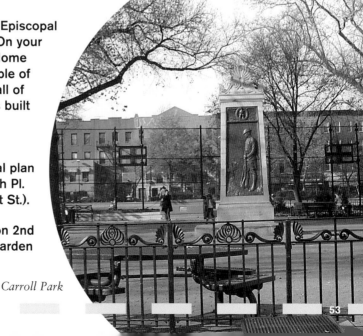

*Carroll Park*

- Turn right on Smith, where elementary schoolers have painted images of peace and harmony in murals on your right. When the Gowanus Canal was thriving commercially, this was a strip of taverns and rooming houses.

- Turn right on 4th Pl. and pass under the train trestle for a final stroll through the exceptional residential layout of Carroll Gardens.

- Turn left at Court and conclude your walk with some refreshment at the oldest bar in Brooklyn, P.J. Hanley's. It was sold in 2005 by the Hanley family, who had owned it since 1958, but the bar had operated under other names since 1874.

- Walk back to Smith and 2nd for the F or G train, or board the B75 bus on Smith for a ride along Brooklyn's "restaurant row" to Bergen St. and transfer to the subway there. If you're going to dine, get off the bus when you see what you like, be it French, Asian, Italian, Caribbean, or inventive American/Continental.

## DINING across THE HIGHWAY

The wedge between Hicks St. and the waterfront is theoretically the west side of Carroll Gardens—or Cobble Hill, if you're north of Kane St.—but its identity is murky because the Brooklyn-Queens Expressway sequesters it from the rest of the neighborhood (pedestrians can cross only at Sackett, Union, and Summit Sts.). Some give the area its own name, the Columbia St. district, while others place it in Red Hook, though Hamilton Ave. farther south is often considered the Red Hook border. Identity crisis and semi-isolation notwithstanding, a few acclaimed restaurants draw diners. Located on Union St. between Hicks and Columbia for over a century, Ferdinando's (718-855-1545) specializes in real Sicilian fare like pasta con sarde (sardines) and caponatina, an eggplant appetizer. Across the street, five-year-old Schnäck (718-855-2879) serves up addictively sized and sauced mini-burgers and other comfort food with an edge in a colorful, kitschy, and ultracasual setting. Alma (718-643-5400), which opened in 2002 at Columbia and DeGraw, offers sophisticated Mexican cuisine and a view of Lower Manhattan (across a still-active Brooklyn shipyard) from both its second-story dining room and rooftop patio.

# POINTS OF INTEREST

**Brooklyn Lyceum** 227 4th Ave., Brooklyn, NY 11215, 866-GOWANUS

**Canal Bar** 270 3rd Ave., Brooklyn, NY 11215, 718-246-0011

**Issue Project Room** 400 Carroll St., Brooklyn, NY 11231, 718-330-0313

**Gowanus Dredgers** 2nd St. at Gowanus Canal, Brooklyn, NY 11231, 718-243-0849

**gallerythe.org** 343 Smith St., Brooklyn, NY 11231

**Carroll Park** Smith and President Sts., Brooklyn, NY 11231

**P.J. Hanley's** 449 Court St., Brooklyn, NY 11231, 718-834-8223

# ROUTE SUMMARY

1.  Begin on 4th Ave. at President St. and walk south.
2.  Turn right on Carroll St.
3.  Turn right on 3rd Ave.
4.  Turn left on President, then left on Nevins St.
5.  Turn right on Carroll and cross the Gowanus Canal.
6.  Turn left on Bond St., then left on 2nd St.
7.  Go back to Bond and make a right.
8.  Turn left on 1st St.
9.  Turn right on Hoyt St., left on Carroll, and right on Smith St.
10. Enter and exit Carroll Park on President, then go left.
11. Turn left on Clinton St.
12. Turn left on 1st Pl.
13. Turn right on Court St., then left on 2nd Pl.
14. Turn right on Smith.
15. Turn right on 4th Pl.
16. Turn left on Court.
17. Return to Smith and 2nd for subway or bus.

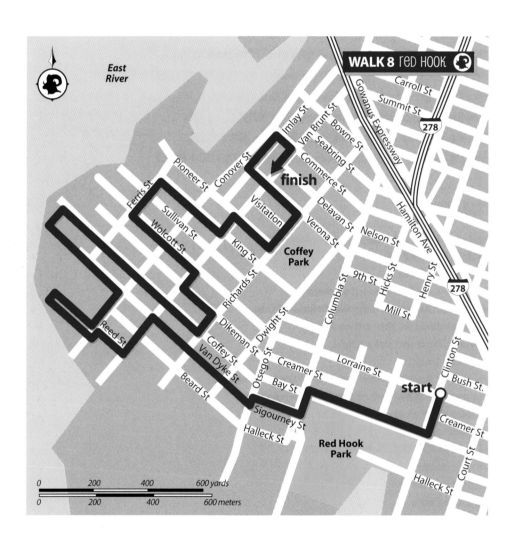

East River

WALK 8 red HOOK

Carroll St
Summit St
278

Imlay St
Van Brunt St
Bowne St
Seabring St
Commerce St

Gowanus Expressway

Pioneer St
Conover St

Ferris St

finish

Visitation

Delavan St
Verona St

Hamilton Ave

Sullivan St
Wolcott St

King St

Nelson St

Coffey Park

9th St
Hicks St
Henry St

Richards St

Columbia St

Mill St

278

Reed St

Dwight St

Dikeman St

Coffey St
Van Dyke St

Otsego St

Creamer St

Lorraine St

Clinton St
Bush St.

start

Beard St

Bay St

Sigourney St

Creamer St

Halleck St

Red Hook Park

Court St

Halleck St

0       200       400       600 yards
0       200       400       600 meters

# 8 reD HOOK: reinventing a SHIPPING OUTPOST

**BOUNDARIES: Clinton St., Reed St., Valentino Pier, Commerce St.**
**DISTANCE: Approx. 3 miles**
**SUBWAY: F to Smith–9 St., transfer to B77 bus to Red Hook**

Red Hook is the overnight success of Brooklyn's renaissance. In a matter of months the neighborhood went from off-the-radar rat hole to purported hotbed of gentrification and fine cuisine. But the hype was probably premature. Cruise-ship passengers disembarking at Red Hook's new terminal won't be converted into tourists if their perception of Brooklyn is based on the immediate vicinity of the terminal. And while Van Brunt St. now sports two well-received upscale restaurants, the Good Fork and 360, that doesn't really justify a "restaurant row" coronation. Furthermore, Red Hook will likely never be able to shed its accessibility problem: the nearest subway station is a 20-minute walk. Still, the neighborhood has been garnering more attention in the past few years than in the previous 60. The 1946 construction of the Gowanus Expressway basically cut off Red Hook from the rest of Brooklyn. Around the same time, the shipping trade started to drop off. The wharves and warehouses left behind are now among the area's prime attractions, along with cobblestone streets, parks, and a funky artistic vibe. And somehow, Red Hook's coarse past—Al Capone started here and these streets inspired such hardscrabble tales as *Last Exit to Brooklyn* and *A View from the Bridge*—is part of the appeal too.

● Get off the bus at Clinton and Lorraine Sts., cross Lorraine, and walk south on Clinton. At Bay St., turn right. Expansive Red Hook Park opens up before you on your left. On your right is Sol Goldman Pool, a Works Progress Administration project nearly as large as four Olympic-sized pools. Beyond the pool you can see Red Hook Housing, one of the oldest and largest public-housing complexes in the city (over two-thirds of Red Hook's population live there). It was built during the Depression for dock workers and their families but gained notoriety in the late 20th century as drugs and crime ran rampant.

● Turn left on Columbia St., then right on Sigourney St. and left on Otsego St. to walk around the Red Hook Community Farm. Opened in 2003 where a rundown playground used to be, the farm is tended by young people who receive job training and education in farming and food service. The produce is sold to local restaurants, donated to the needy, and offered for sale to the public at the garden on Saturdays and in nearby Coffey Park on Wednesdays.

● From Otsego, turn right on Van Dyke St. and walk one skeevy block to Dwight St., where you'll find the Liberty Heights Tap Room. Ales are made on-site (there's a brewery tour on Saturdays) and in the summer can be enjoyed on a roof deck. Look down Dwight to your left—the next intersection, with Beard St., was approximately the site of Fort Defiance, a Revolutionary War post destroyed by the British in September 1776.

● Continue on Van Dyke to see some classic brick buildings—#66, with its iron-railed stoop and wooden door, is a particular beaut—as well as the rehabbed plant of Red Hand Compositions, now housing a technology firm.

● When you cross Richards St., you've entered the part of Red Hook known as the Back. Extending to the river, this west side of Red Hook is where most revitalization has occurred. On your right past Richards, the gray fortresslike 1859 storehouse of the Brooklyn Clay Retort and Fire Brick Works has gained city landmark status. Across the street, another manufacturing relic is noteworthy for its tall brick chimney.

● The next street is Van Brunt, commercial hub of the neighborhood. Turn left and you'll soon approach the biggest commercial enterprise in the area, the 52,000-square-foot Fairway supermarket that opened in early 2006 in a Civil War–era coffee warehouse. Turn right on Reed St. and, across from the Fairway parking lot, you can't miss the private house at #26, ostentatiously adorned with patriotic and nautical items, mostly salvaged by a garbageman friend of the homeowner.

● Turn left on Conover St. and use the sidewalk inside the parking lot to your right to reach the Garden Pier—a swath of urban beautification at its most effective. This was a dumping ground just a decade ago! Follow the path on the right onto a charming esplanade. Walk to the end on the paved lane, then come back via the wood-planked side. Continue to the Waterfront Museum, located inside a 1914 Lehigh Valley Railroad barge and offering maritime exhibits, music, and circus shows. Go to the end of the pier where the barge is moored for dynamite views of the Verrazano-Narrows

Bridge and Lady Liberty. The neighboring piers are the only remaining warehouse piers from Brooklyn's industrial heyday, when the waterfront all the way north to Queens was lined with such wharves. To your left is the Beard Street Warehouse, now filled with art/design studios and offices.

● Go back to Conover St., turn left and walk toward the generic BAR sign hanging from a building on your right. This is Sunny's, the sole surviving longshoremen's bar. Vintage kitchenwares are on display, including the huge coffeepots where workers used to fill up for their morning jolt. But Sunny's—which has been in the same family for generations—supports Red Hook's present-day population too, with art exhibits and book readings.

● At the Conover/Van Dyke intersection, where a ginormous satellite TV tower threatens to obliterate the historic ambience, turn left. Enter Pier 41 and go left into the parking lot. Look for the yellow door with the sign PIES HERE. Steve's Authentic Key Lime Pies uses only fresh-squeezed key limes, and the mini-pie or chocolate-coated frozen pie on a stick is a good refresher for your walk.

● Return to Van Dyke and make a left. Walk through the parking lot at Ferris St. to reach Valentino Pier. Popular for fishing and sunset gazing, the former Pier 39 is the closest you can get to the Statue of Liberty on land, and its overall pleasantness—including the lawn between the pier and street—is one of NYC's best-kept secrets.

● Leave the pier near the flagpole and turn right on Coffey St., walking past several nice brick homes. At the corner with Conover, note the original street name—PARTITION STREET—on the

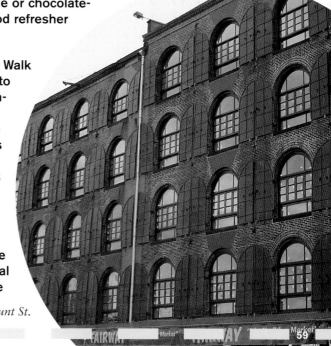

*480–500 Van Brunt St.*

building to your left, between the second and third floors. The street was rechristened in honor of influential 19th-century politician Michael Joseph Coffey, who served the area for over 30 years until he ran afoul of Brooklyn's corrupt Democratic Party machine.

- On the other side of Conover, 128 Coffey St. has lion's heads on its mahogany doors. This 1910 building was elegantly restored in 2005 and sits across from a considerably more modern-looking building, with its slanted skylight roof and heavily windowed façade.

- Proceed on cobblestone Coffey across Van Brunt. This is one of Red Hook's more attractive blocks, thanks in part to flowerpots on the stoops. The household at #94A, on your left, has gone all out decorating their front yard—colored lights, birdhouses, flowers real and artificial, even a waterfall are involved.

- Turn left on Richards, another pretty block. Then go left on Dikeman St. and right on Van Brunt. Baked, located on your right, opened in 2004—soon after 360 and not long before the Good Fork—setting up Red Hook as an epicurean destination. Their irresistible cakes feature buttercream frosting in flavors like Grand Marnier and cinnamon, with toppings like pistachios and pralines. A couple of doors down, the Kentler International Drawing Space showcases contemporary works on paper.

- Turn left on Wolcott St. and see a Pentecostal church and houses beyond it with roof patios. The Good Shepherd center is a more notable newbie on your left at Conover. Containing an alternative high school and social services, this was the first new building to open in Red Hook (in May 2001) in many years, and its boat shape is a nod to the area's heritage.

- Proceed on Wolcott to Ferris and turn right, walking along the perimeter of a great complex of brick buildings. After the next street, Sullivan (there's no sign), look to Red Hook's new wave of shipping—cruise shipping, that is. In April 2006 the $52 million Brooklyn Cruise Terminal at Pier 12 became a home port for the *Queen Mary 2* and for Princess and Carnival ships. The terminal is located within the Atlantic Basin, which was the United States' largest port facility in the 19th century.

*Valentino Pier*

- Turn right on King St. and walk past Red Hook in progress—several industrial buildings in assorted states of neglect or rehabilitation.

- Turn left when you reach Van Brunt. At the corner with Pioneer St., a bar called the Red Hook Bait & Tackle Shop Fishing Club is decorated à la a hunting lodge. Next door, the Old Pioneer Bar keeps its kitsch out front: benches affixed with license plates from every state. The Pioneer is known for its barbecue and its beer garden.

- Turn right on Pioneer. Classy brick homes with rose bushes share this tree-lined block with drab housing and industrial conversions. The building at #111 is known as the Smo~King Church, a conflation of its past inhabitants—the Norwegian Seaman's Church, which built the property in 1878 and stayed for about 50 years, and Smo~King Products, manufacturer of ashtrays and barbecues, which moved in afterward. The current tenant makes robotic sculptures and exhibits various artists' work. The street becomes less desirable on your right as you approach Richards.

- Turn left on Richards and walk alongside Coffey Park. Between Visitation Pl. and Verona St. rises the Visitation of the Blessed Virgin Mary church, featuring a vaulted wooden ceiling and Tiffany stained-glass windows.

- Go left on Verona to Imlay St. and turn right for one last glimpse of Red Hook's glory days: the huge warehouses of the New York Dock Company that resemble either a castle or a jail. The iron balconies were unusual for industrial architecture.

- Turn right between the buildings onto Commerce St., then turn right on Van Brunt and enjoy the variously painted or bricked façades on your right. The blue building with a gas pump out front is the RSA Diesel Gallery, a venue for alternative art and performances.

- Cross Van Brunt and take the B61 bus to Jay St.–Borough Hall for the A, C, or F train.

## POINTS OF INTEREST

**Red Hook Community Farm** Columbia and Sigourney Sts., Brooklyn, NY 11231

**Liberty Heights Tap Room** 34 Van Dyke St., Brooklyn, NY 11231, 718-246-8050

**Fairway of Red Hook** 480–500 Van Brunt St., Brooklyn, NY 11231, 718-694-6868

**Garden Pier** Conover and Beard Sts., Brooklyn, NY 11231

**Waterfront Museum** 290 Conover St., Brooklyn, NY 11231, 718-624-4719

**Sunny's** 253 Conover St., Brooklyn, NY 11231, 718-625-8211

**Steve's Authentic Key Lime Pies** Pier 41/204 Van Dyke St., Brooklyn, NY 11231, 718-858-5333

**Valentino Pier** Coffey and Ferris Sts., Brooklyn, NY 11231

**Baked** 359 Van Brunt St., Brooklyn, NY 11231, 718-222-0345

**Kentler International Drawing Space** 353 Van Brunt St., Brooklyn, NY 11231, 718-875-2098

**Red Hook Bait & Tackle Shop Fishing Club** 320 Van Brunt St., Brooklyn, NY 11231, 718-797-4892

**Old Pioneer Bar** 318 Van Brunt St., Brooklyn, NY 11231, 718-624-0700

**Coffey Park** Richards and Verona Sts., Brooklyn, NY 11231

**RSA Diesel Gallery** 242 Van Brunt St., Brooklyn, NY 11231, 917-251-4070

# route summary

1. Begin at Clinton and Lorraine Sts. Walk south on Clinton and turn right on Bay St.
2. Turn left on Columbia St.
3. Turn right on Sigourney St. and left on Otsego St.
4. Turn right on Van Dyke St.
5. Turn left on Van Brunt St., then right on Reed St.
6. Turn left on Conover St. and go right onto the pier.
7. From the pier, go left on Conover.
8. Go left on Van Dyke to Pier 41 and then to Valentino Pier.
9. From Valentino Pier, turn right on Coffey St.
10. Turn left on Richards St., left on Dikeman St., and right on Van Brunt.
11. Turn left on Wolcott St.
12. Turn right on Ferris St.
13. Turn right on King St.
14. Turn left on Van Brunt.
15. Turn right on Pioneer St.
16. Turn left on Richards.
17. Turn left on Verona St. and right on Imlay St.
18. Turn right on Commerce St.
19. Turn right on Van Brunt and take the bus to the subway.

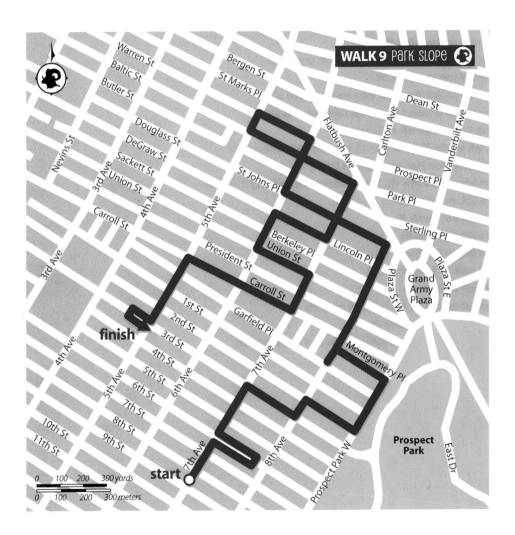

Warren St
Baltic St
Butler St
Bergen St
St Marks Pl
Dean St
Carlton Ave
Vanderbilt Ave
Prospect Pl
Park Pl
Flatbush Ave
Douglass St
DeGraw St
Sackett St
Nevins St
3rd Ave
Union St
4th Ave
St Johns Pl
Carroll St
5th Ave
Sterling Pl
3rd Ave
President St
Berkeley Pl
Union St
Lincoln Pl
Plaza St W
Plaza St E
Grand
Army
Plaza
Carroll St
1st St
2nd St
Garfield Pl
**finish**
3rd St
4th St
4th Ave
5th St
6th St
5th Ave
6th Ave
7th St
7th Ave
8th St
9th St
10th St
11th St
Montgomery Pl
**Prospect
Park**
East Dr
7th Ave
8th Ave
Prospect Park W
**start**

0    100    200    300 yards
0    100    200    300 meters

# 9 Park Slope: The Gold Coast Still Glitters

BOUNDARIES: **9th St., 5th Ave., Prospect Pl., Prospect Park W.**
DISTANCE: **Approx. 3½ miles**
SUBWAY: **F to 7th Ave.**

Park Slope was rediscovered during the brownstone revival of the late 1960s, so it has been a primo address for some time. The millionaires who transformed it into Brooklyn's Gold Coast after Prospect Park and the Brooklyn Bridge opened in the late 1800s left behind a dazzling array of mansions and townhouses in Romanesque, Queen Anne, Italianate, and Renaissance Revival styles. That classic Brooklyn image of brownstone rowhouses with stoops is found on street after street of Park Slope. Brooklyn also gained its reputation as the "city of churches" from neighborhoods like this. The latter-day citizenry has made it a neighborhood of coffeehouses, wine shops, yoga studios, and boutiques for pampering pets or children. Park Slopers tend to be liberal, white, married, with kids and a dog. A lot of writers live here too. Some have likened Park Slope to a college town. Some have compared it to Paris. Others just think of it as one of America's Victorian treasures.

- **Walk north on 7th Ave. to 7th St. for All Saints Episcopal Church, an 1892 giant boasting Moorish towers within a Romanesque design. A totally different tower rises from Greenwood Baptist Church at the corner of 6th St.**

- **Turn right on 6th St. Methodist Hospital on your right has a place in global and local history. Its worldwide significance is explained in a plaque on your right before you reach the front doors. Then enter the hospital and go into its Phillips Chapel, located off the lobby. Immediately to your left, coins are affixed to a plaque on the wall. They were the pocket change of Stephen Baltz, an 11-year-old passenger aboard a United flight that crashed into the streets of Park Slope on December 16, 1960, while trying to make an emergency landing in Prospect Park. Young Stephen died in the hospital the next day. All the other victims, including two men who were selling Christmas trees on the sidewalk, were pronounced dead at the scene.**

- **Go back to 7th Ave. and turn right. The handsome school that sprawls from 5th to 4th Sts. on your right was once Manual Training High School, which graduated yukmeister**

Henny Youngman, six-time Oscar nominee Thelma Ritter, and the 1944 Nobel laureate in physics, Isidor Isaac Rabi. It later changed its name to John Jay High School, and in the 1980s and '90s deteriorated—as Park Slope grew more and more affluent—into one of the worst schools in the city. On your left past 4th St. is the Cocoa Bar, one of several eateries remaking Brooklyn into a chocoholic's haven. They make candies that coat chocolate over such fillings as strawberry shortcake, peanut butter and jelly, and Kahlua with marshmallow and cookie, as well as concoctions in a cup like the Chocolatte.

● Turn right on 3rd St., then go left at 8th Ave. The first house on your left looks like it was designed for the country instead of the city. It was built in 1913 by the Neergaard family, who founded a Park Slope pharmacy in 1888 that's still in business. At the next corner, the august Byzantine Melkite Catholic Church of the Virgin Mary has been a house of worship for Christians of Arab descent since 1952. It was constructed in 1903 for Congregationalists.

● Go right on 2nd St. If you've seen *The Wizard of Oz,* talking trees are old hat. But how about a tree that speaks sign language? Look in front of #646 on your right.

● On Prospect Park W., 2nd St. is flanked by two designs by William Tubby, a favorite architect of Brooklyn's smart set at the turn of the century. William Childs, founder of the Bon Ami scouring powder brand, hired Tubby in 1900 to build his mansion at #53 and again in 1910 for the house at #61 that Childs gave his daughter as a wedding present. Theodore Roosevelt, a friend of Childs's, may have been an overnight guest at #53. The Ethical Culture Society, which occupies the Childs house, used to run a school in the gigantic 1889 mansion next door. Today it's Poly Prep Lower School. This Victorian-era beauty can play tricks on your eyes: it looks symmetrical at first glance, but the tower on the left is smaller and rounded compared to the polygonal right tower, and the doors are skewed to the left. Ahead, down Prospect Park W., you can see the Soldiers' and Sailors' Memorial Arch in Grand Army Plaza. The limestone Renaissance palace at #28 with lions and other embellishment was designed in 1901 by Charles Brigham, who worked mostly in Boston.

● Turn left on Montgomery Pl., which one architectural historian has described as a "great urban ensemble." The initial development in 1888 comprised about 20 houses, including all those on your left from #36 to #60. They launched the career of their 24-year-old architect, Charles P.H. Gilbert, who went on to design several mansions on 5th Ave. in Manhattan. Other architects were responsible for later houses on Montgomery.

- Go left on 8th Ave. to Garfield Pl., where the two buildings of Congregation Beth Elohim stand across from each other: the domed Neoclassical synagogue on your near left and the Art Deco–ish temple house opposite it. Moses stands atop the corner of the temple house with the Ten Commandments.

- Turn around and walk north on 8th Ave. Some of the spectacular mansions here should be seen from the side street as well as the avenue, such as the reddish-brown behemoth on your right at Carroll St., which could be called the house that Chiclets built (because the gum inventor lived here). It is supposedly haunted by servants who died in its elevator after it malfunctioned. A couple of doors down 8th on the right, a Montessori school occupies a former private home, built in 1916, that looks like it was imported from the English countryside. The elegant apartment building next to it was also built as a single-family home, in 1909, for a brewery executive. The grande dame of Park Slope is the Montauk Club on your right at Lincoln Pl. If this Victorian Gothic Venetian palazzo doesn't convince you of the club's wealth and prestige, consider that Brooklyn may have remained an independent city if it weren't for club members, who are believed to have swayed the close public vote in favor of consolidation with Manhattan. The lower frieze on the building depicts the club's founders laying the cornerstone; the higher, wraparound frieze illustrates Montauk Indian history. There's still

*Montauk Club*

a club inside, but membership is no longer exclusionary. The top floors have been turned over to apartments.

● Turn left on St. John's Pl. Watch on your right for the flying buttresses of Grace United Methodist Church. It's diagonally across 7th from Memorial Presbyterian, which has Tiffany stained-glass windows. Both of these Gothic churches were built in the 1880s. St. John's Episcopal, on your right after crossing 7th, was started earlier: its chapel and rectory date to 1870. Also in the Gothic vernacular, St. John's is enhanced by a garden. Across the street, note the red gable embossed with a caduceus, the intertwining-snakes symbol of the medical profession. The first owner of this house, in 1888, was a doctor.

● Turn right on 6th Ave. St. Augustine's, on the left at Sterling, is considered the masterpiece of the Parfitt Brothers, who designed a number of illustrious Brooklyn churches, including Grace United. Towers, spires, and lancet windows abound in this phenomenal church, which is crowned with a copper statue of the angel Gabriel blowing his trumpet.

● Go left on Prospect Pl. for a charming assemblage of Queen Anne houses from the 1880s on your left at #54–#64.

● At 5th Ave., cross over to the Chocolate Room, another of Brooklyn's cacao-fueled emporiums, acclaimed for its chocolate layer cake, hot chocolate, and fresh-mint chip ice cream. Walk one block south on 5th Ave. to Park Pl. and turn left. On your right after 6th, the barnlike residence at #90 used to be a carriage house for a mansion on the avenue. All these matching townhouses down the right side are brownstones—despite their varying hues—and they're some of the earliest in the Slope. The ones with bay windows from #100 to #116 were built in the 1870s, and many of those with flat fronts date to 1868.

● Turn right on 7th Ave. On your right, #8–#16 are among the first rowhouses in Park Slope, constructed around 1860 (and obviously since restored). On your left at Sterling Pl., a delightful oriel protrudes from the corner mansion, once home to the Canadian opera star Lillian Ward. The Ward mansion was miraculously spared serious damage by the United crash in 1960, which occurred at its doorstep. A church

*3rd St. brownstones*

kitty-corner from the mansion was destroyed, and you can still tell where the apartment house at 126 Sterling Pl., a few doors off 7th, was repaired after being struck—bricks above the top windows are a different color from those below. Continuing along 7th, Ozzie's coffeehouse on your left at Lincoln has preserved the old-timey or vintage interior from when it was a pharmacy. Across the avenue is the 110-year-old Brooklyn Conservatory of Music.

● Turn right on Lincoln Pl. The 1887 Romanesque mansion on your right at #153 just became a condominium. Prior to the conversion, it somehow had been left alone for over 40 years—while the neighborhood filled with wealth and children—even though everyone knew a hot-sheet hotel was operating inside. (One tryst ended in murder in 1999, when a woman was hanged from the shower rod by her lover.) The Baptist church on your right at 6th was designed by the architect of the Lillian Ward house. This church came first, in 1880, and had a steeple rising from its corner section until the fourth-deadliest hurricane in U.S. history, nicknamed the Long Island Express, barreled through in September 1938.

● Go left on 6th and then left on Union St. The Park Slope Food Coop, on your right, started back before terms like "organic" and "macrobiotic" became part of everyone's dietary lexicon. Now in its fourth decade, it's the largest member-owned grocery in the country. It's next to Squad 1, an elite rescue unit of the Fire Department of New York that lost 12 men on 9/11. Across Union, a three-sided mural brightens an industrial building.

- Turn right on 7th. The Old First Reformed Church on your right at Carroll St. serves a congregation established in the 17th century that has had four previous homes around Brooklyn.

- Go right on Carroll. Recycling gets a pretty face from the floral collage on your left that was created from food packaging by local second graders.

- At 5th Ave., turn left. Many of these bistros and boutiques have sprouted up in the past decade. Into the 1990s, 5th was still mostly a working-class Latino strip, outside of yuppies' shopping and dining territory.

- Turn right at 3rd St. Enter J.J. Byrne Park and proceed to the Old Stone House, a 1930s replica of the Dutch farmhouse that was constructed about 100 feet to the east in 1699. On August 27, 1776, beginning around 2:00 A.M., a volunteer regiment of 400 Marylanders engaged a much larger force of British and Hessian soldiers in a battle at the house, which was held by the British during the war. It was a tactical maneuver to allow the Continental Army to evacuate Brooklyn. The diversion succeeded and the other troops made it to Manhattan, but nearly 300 of the Maryland men were killed. Their sacrifice is commemorated in a museum exhibit inside the Old Stone House. As if that's not enough history, these grounds would also become the first home field of the baseball team eventually known as the Brooklyn Dodgers, who played at Byrne Park's previous incarnation, Washington Park, starting around 1894.

- Cross 5th Ave. and take the Cobble Hill–bound B63 bus to the Atlantic Ave./Pacific St. station, which is served by 10 subway lines.

## POINTS OF INTEREST

**Cocoa Bar** 228 7th Ave., Brooklyn, NY 11215, 718-499-4080

**The Chocolate Room** 86 5th Ave., Brooklyn, NY 11217, 718-783-2900

**Ozzie's** 57 7th Ave., Brooklyn, NY 11215, 718-398-6695

**J.J. Byrne Park** 3rd St. and 5th Ave., Brooklyn, NY 11215

**Old Stone House** J.J. Byrne Park, 3rd St. and 5th Ave., Brooklyn, NY 11215, 718-768-3195

# route summary

1. Begin at 7th Ave. and walk north from 9th St.
2. Go right on 6th St. to Methodist Hospital.
3. Return to 7th Ave. and turn right to resume walking north.
4. Turn right on 3rd St., then left at 8th Ave.
5. Turn right on 2nd St.
6. Turn left on Prospect Park W.
7. Turn left on Montgomery Pl.
8. Go left on 8th to Garfield Pl., then turn around.
9. From 8th, turn left on St. John's Pl.
10. Turn right on 6th Ave.
11. Go left on Prospect Pl.
12. Turn left on 5th Ave., then left on Park Pl.
13. Turn right on 7th.
14. Turn right on Lincoln Pl.
15. Go left on 6th, then left on Union St.
16. Turn right on 7th.
17. Go right on Carroll St.
18. Turn left on 5th Ave.
19. Go right on 3rd St. to the Old Stone House.
20. Go back to 5th Ave. and take the B63 bus to the Atlantic Ave./Pacific St. subway.

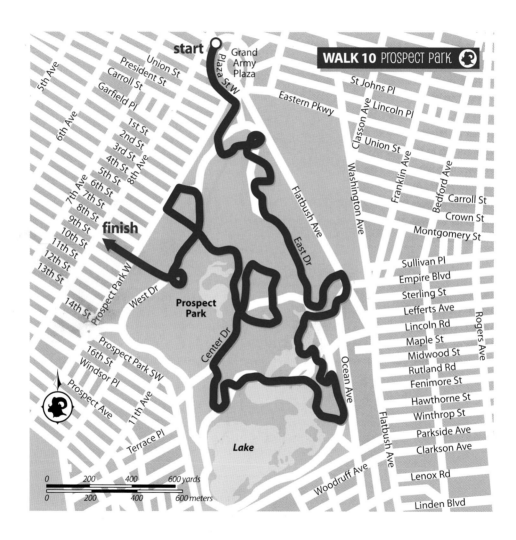

start

Grand
Army
Plaza

Union St
President St
Carroll St
Garfield Pl

5th Ave
6th Ave

1st St
2nd St
3rd St
4th St
5th St
6th St
7th St
8th St
9th St
10th St
11th St
12th St
13th St
14th St

4th Ave
8th Ave
7th Ave

finish

Plaza St W

St Johns Pl
Eastern Pkwy
Lincoln Pl
Union St

Classon Ave
Washington Ave
Franklin Ave
Bedford Ave

Carroll St
Crown St
Montgomery St

Flatbush Ave
East Dr

Sullivan Pl
Empire Blvd
Sterling St
Lefferts Ave
Lincoln Rd
Maple St
Midwood St
Rutland Rd
Fenimore St
Hawthorne St
Winthrop St
Parkside Ave
Clarkson Ave

Rogers Ave

Prospect Park W
West Dr

**Prospect
Park**

Center Dr
Ocean Ave
Flatbush Ave

Prospect Park SW
16th St
Windsor Pl
11th Ave
Terrace Pl

Prospect Ave

*Lake*

Woodruff Ave
Lenox Rd
Linden Blvd

0    200    400    600 yards
0    200    400    600 meters

# 10 Prospect Park: Jewel in the Crown

**BOUNDARIES:** **Flatbush Ave., Ocean Ave., Prospect Park Lake, Prospect Park W.**
**DISTANCE:** **Approx. 4 miles**
**SUBWAY:** **2 or 3 to Grand Army Plaza**

Frederick Law Olmsted and Calvert Vaux, pioneers of landscape architecture and the urban parks movement in the United States, are most famous for Central Park but were prouder of Prospect Park. When they had designed Central Park a decade earlier, they were frustrated by certain restrictions, such as the required rectangular shape. Freed of such constraints for Prospect Park, nature-loving Olmsted and Vaux created a park they considered more naturalistic. Before construction commenced in the 1860s, Brooklynites had only Green-Wood Cemetery and 30-acre Washington (Fort Greene) Park for a bucolic escape. By the time Prospect Park was completed in 1873, they would find within its 526 acres a natural forest, meadows, rolling hills, and a series of waterways coursing through the eastern half and emptying into a lake. The park also contains some notable statuary and architecture, as well as historic and recreational accoutrements ranging from solemn war memorials to a Children's Corner complete with a zoo and carousel.

- From the subway, walk on Plaza St. W. to the main entrance of Prospect Park, heralded by four eagle-topped columns. Follow the path between the two eagle columns on the right. Take either path around the oval grove, go to your left after the downward slope, and walk through Meadowport Arch, which was created by Olmsted and has a double opening onto Long Meadow.

- Go to the left. The trees on your left form the 9/11 Grove, where candlelight vigils were held following the tragedy and trees have been planted in memory of the victims. Take one of the dirt paths uphill through the grove and onto pavement. Go right, and walk with the 9/11 Grove on your right and a full view of the Grand Army Plaza arch on your left.

- Immediately after passing where wooden barriers line both sides of the drive, take the narrower paved path between trees on your left. Go left again to continue downhill, then make yet another left at the bottom to walk under Endale Arch. This is

Brooklyn's oldest bridge, still standing from when the park was created in 1867. Its name was compressed from "enter dale," which is what you do as you come out the other side at the edge of Long Meadow.

● Go to your left, then up the concrete staircase on your left, and cross East Dr. Go left and proceed to the broad steps on your right leading into the Rose Garden, a part of the Vale of Cashmere where roses cannot grow because the soil is not deep enough. Go down the steps to a large, shallow, empty oval pool. Go to your left and you'll pass two more pools—similar shape, similarly empty. It has nothing to do with the time of year. The pipes feeding these pools leaked on their opening day in 1969 and flooded the area. The pools were never filled again. Perhaps because these fountains are unused, the Vale of Cashmere is one of the less visited areas of the park. And perhaps because of the resultant low traffic, it has had an iffy reputation. So be alert . . . and also be ready for one of the park's best-kept secrets. Go to your right after the third pool, then down the path to your right, and you'll enter a lovely secluded oasis where the fountains *do* work. Here, sequestered from the bustle of urban life, you can lose yourself in the beauty and tranquility of nature, just as Olmsted and Vaux desired.

● Walk all the way around—just follow the red-brick road—and after passing another fountain take the blacktop path on the left. Stay on it with Nellie's Lawn on your right. At an opening between trees, cross the lawn and turn left onto East Dr. Three historic markers appear in quick succession. First, watch on your left for a boulder beside a tree identifying the Continental Army's line of defense during the Battle of Long Island. Then, on your right, another boulder bears a plaque that explains why this part of the park is known as Battle Pass. Continuing on East Dr., just before the traffic light, you'll find on your left an eagle monument where an oak tree was cut down and thrown in the way of advancing British troops.

● Stay on East Dr. When it diverges from the sidewalk path, take the path and follow it right up to the carousel. Built in 1912, the carousel was moved into the park from—where else?—Coney Island and has been splendidly restored over the past two decades. Another transplant is the wooden kiosk with an up-pointing arrow on its red roof, located across from the carousel. This is a tollbooth from the old Flatbush

Turnpike, later replaced by Flatbush Ave. The old Dutch farmhouse next to the carousel was also relocated from Flatbush Ave., where it was constructed in the 1780s. The Lefferts House now serves as a free living-history museum. The path between the farmhouse and the carousel leads to the Prospect Park Zoo.

- From in front of the carousel, take the path farther from the Lefferts House, then turn right onto the blacktop drive. When it splits, go to your right, cross the drive, and follow the path on the left (next to a water fountain) toward the woods. After the path changes from gravel to paved, go to your left and down the steps. At the next fork, go right and cross Binnen Bridge, named for the Binnenwater that flows beneath it (*binnen* is Dutch for "within"). That's a lily pond on your right.

- On the other side of the bridge, follow the path to your left down to the viewing platform. The Beaux Arts Boathouse, modeled on the Sansoviniana library in St. Mark's square in Venice, was built in 1905. By 1960, the Boathouse had been neglected so badly that it was targeted for demolition. But it was saved by a citizens' campaign and is now on the National Register of Historic Places and the city's landmarks roster.

- Facing the Boathouse, go to your right, walking beside the Lullwater. Go up the log staircase and go left to reach Lullwater Bridge, another good place to photograph the Boathouse. Note the rustic shelter across the water to your right—seven of them were recently erected in the park, reintroducing a feature from the Olmsted/ Vaux plan. The shelters were made as the original ones had been—no nails, only pegs and dowels holding the logs together. Proceed across the bridge to the Boathouse so you can

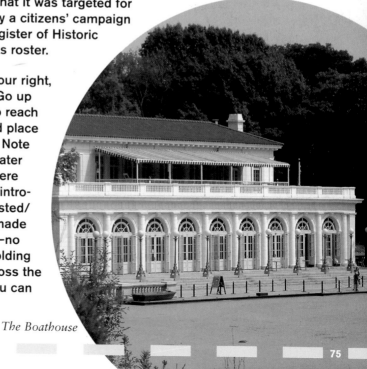

*The Boathouse*

see its terra cotta detail close-up. Go inside for the nature-themed exhibits of the first urban Audubon Center in the country (Prospect Park was an apt choice, as it's home to some 260 species of birds).

- Leave the Boathouse on the side where you entered, but follow the path to your left. Not far along on your left is the squat and gnarly Camperdown Elm, planted in 1872 and now protected by a fence. There are fewer than 10 such trees in the world—Mr. Camperdown made just a handful of cuttings of his elm in Scotland that, due to a mutation, grew low and parallel to the ground instead of up. Like the Boathouse, this tree was once slated for removal. Preservation efforts for both were led by poet and Brooklyn resident/booster Marianne Moore, who penned an ode to the elm.

- Head over to the Cleft Ridge Span. This was the last of the park's bridges to be built, and it had to be done on the cheap because the city was in a financial crisis in the early 1870s. But the cast concrete used instead of more expensive cut stone later became common in bridge construction around the country. After the bridge, go right and walk to the Oriental Pavilion ahead on your left, reconstructed after a 1974 fire consumed everything but the cast-iron pillars.

- Down the steps, follow the path to your right to walk around the Concert Grove and its busts of composers. After Mozart and Beethoven, you'll come to Irish bard Thomas Moore, who penned the poem ("Lalla Rookh") that mentions a "vale of Cashmere." After passing Grieg, go down the steps to another bust, that of Washington Irving, native New Yorker and author of "The Legend of Sleepy Hollow." Facing Irving (the first bust ever installed in the park), turn right and proceed to the Imagination Playground, where another local writer is honored: Ezra Jack Keats, the award-winning children's book author who was born and raised in Brooklyn. Peter and his dog Willie, two of Keats's recurring characters, are represented, and other imagination-stimulating objects also inhabit the playground.

- Come out of the playground and turn left, walking on the path along East Dr. When you reach the Drummer's Grove on your left (created after a West Indian drumming circle had been meeting at the spot for years), walk across the lawn opposite it to the lake, all 60 acres of which were dug with picks and shovels during the park's construction. Off to the right is a World War I memorial listing Brooklyn's casualties. Loss

## MUSIC IN THE air

It should be no surprise that a place that produced the likes of George Gershwin, Beverly Sills, Carole King, and Jay-Z enjoys making music and making a special occasion out of it. Every year Brooklyn hosts several music festivals, showcasing a variety of genres and performers from up-and-coming acts to legends. Many of the festivals are held outdoors, and often admission is free.

Celebrate Brooklyn! has been lighting up the Prospect Park Bandshell for nearly 30 years. Running throughout the summer, the festival includes rock, jazz, classical, reggae, funk, folk, Latino, and African concerts, as well as dance and family-oriented performances.

The Red Hook Waterfront Arts Festival is in its second decade of bringing dance and hip-hop to the Beard St. pier for one Saturday in June. The program includes workshops as well as performances. The Brooklyn Hip-Hop Festival, launched in 2005, is staged one day in late June at Dumbo's Empire-Fulton Ferry State Park.

Over in Coney Island, the Village Voice Siren Music Festival is a one-day, two-stage free extravaganza of indie rock. Started in 2001, it takes place in July and draws a couple hundred thousand fans.

A fairly recent addition to Brooklyn's music calendar is the Williamsburg Jazz Festival, which features a week of shows at several different venues. Some concerts are free, others charge a nominal admission. The mid-September festival is preceded by occasional performances during the summer also produced by the Jazz Festival.

rather than heroism sets the mood, accentuated by the veiled angel of death at the center. The honor-roll tablets were crafted by Daniel Chester French, sculptor of the Lincoln Memorial.

● With your back to the memorial, walk straight ahead on the path before you. It curves around to the other side of Wollman Rink and brings you face-to-face with Abraham Lincoln holding the Emancipation Proclamation. This statue, created for the Grand Army Plaza in 1868, was moved into the park in 1895. This spot gives you a feel for what park planners intended for the Concert Grove. People used to sit in the Oriental

Pavilion or on the grass to listen to musicians performing at the lake's edge. That layout was obliterated by the 1950s construction of Wollman Rink, which blocks the view of the lake from the Concert Grove. Fund-raising is under way for replacing Wollman with a Lakeside Center more in keeping with Olmsted and Vaux's vision.

- Turn away from Lincoln and walk to your right, continuing on the next path to the right. Walk uphill into the woods. When you come out on the drive, turn left and cross Terrace Bridge. Beneath you, the Lullwater flows into the lake. Continue to your left.

- Scale Lookout Hill on your right when you see the column with a sphere on top. This monument, believed to be designed by Stanford White, honors the Maryland 400, a volunteer regiment who engaged British soldiers in a skirmish at the nearby Old Stone House to allow evacuation of other Continental troops to Manhattan. The delaying tactic worked, though nearly 300 of the Marylanders were killed.

- Go back down the hill and resume walking in the direction you had been on Wellhouse Dr. The structure that gave the road its name will soon appear on your right. This brick hut, designed by Vaux in 1869, held the pumps that fed the lake from a well 70 feet underground. It became obsolete when the park hooked up to the city's water supply. Just past the Wellhouse is a hilly lawn; walk up it, then go right at the top. When that path forks, go to your left. When you reach the steps that cross the path, turn left and go down them.

- Turn right on Center Dr. Behind the gate on your left you can see some headstones in the Quaker cemetery in existence since before the park was built. It remains property of the Friends Society, so public access is prohibited. Movie star Montgomery Clift is buried there, as are members of the Mott family of applesauce fame.

- Proceed on Center Dr., with the Nethermead field on your right. Look out for the bridge ahead, but do not cross it; instead, just before the bridge, turn onto the path to your left, which leads you down steps. At the bottom, go to the left, then take the first path on your right into the Ravine. Keep walking until you're on Rock Arch Bridge overlooking Ambergill Falls, then go up the steps to your right. At the rustic shelter, turn left and climb more steps, then go to the right, and then to the right again. You're now in the Midwood. Cross Boulder Bridge and turn left. When the path forks, turn right but go down steps on the left side of the path (it's split by some shrubbery). It will bring you to a four-way intersection; go to the right. Continue on this path, cross the drive, then go to the right but stay on the left because the path soon diverges. You want to follow it across Music Grove Bridge and come out in front of the Nethermead, with the Music Pagoda on your left.

- With the bridge/pagoda at your back, turn right. Another waterfall is on your right. Proceed through the Nethermead Arches, which have a stream and a bridle path running beneath them in addition to their pedestrian lane. They are considered the geographic center of the park. You retrace a short stretch you trod earlier, but this time go straight instead of turning into the Ravine. Cross the wooden Esdale Bridge, with falls on your left. Go to your left after the bridge, then make a quick right onto the path through Long Meadow. It takes you to the Picnic House. Walk around to see its impressive front, then keep going straight. Cross West Dr. and go up the steps and to the right. This brings you to Litchfield Villa, the 1857 Italianate mansion of Edwin Litchfield, which you can enter during business hours (the parks department has offices inside). As you walk to the front of the villa, note the corncob capitals on the colonnade between the new annex and the main house. They honor the country's agrarian past and are also found on columns in the U.S. Capitol.

- For a full view of this spectacular mansion, go out of the park at 5th St. and onto Prospect Park W. Turn right and reenter the park at 3rd St. between the two panthers. Note the abandoned stone structure—originally a guardhouse, later a restroom, still unfortunately used as a restroom even without the facilities. Turn right onto West Dr. You'll walk between the Picnic House and Litchfield Villa and pass other administrative buildings on your right. Look out on the left for the Tennis House. From this approach, it will just look like the offices of the Brooklyn Center for the Urban Environment (which it is), but if you walk all the way around it, you'll see it's mostly an open-air structure—and a beautiful one at that. It's sort of a companion piece to the Boathouse, designed a few years later by the same architects in the same Palladian style. The Tennis House was supposed to be a convenience for players of lawn tennis, a sport that was all the rage on the Long Meadow when the building was conceived—but not so popular by the time it was completed. The name stuck, even though the building never really filled its intended purpose. When you're back at the entry gate, go on the path to your left, then take the first path on the right. Cross West Dr. and continue straight on the path. To your left you should see the Bandshell, which features concerts almost every evening in the summer.

● When the path forks, go to the right and exit the park at 9th St. The last monument on your walk is here: Daniel Chester French's bronze relief of the Marquis de Lafayette, who aided the Continental Army during the American Revolution.

● Walk west on 9th St. for one block to the F train.

## POINTS OF INTEREST

**Lefferts Historic House** Near Flatbush Ave. and Empire Blvd., 718-789-2822

**Prospect Park Zoo** Near Flatbush Ave. and Empire Blvd., 718-399-7339

**Audubon Center at the Boathouse** West of Ocean Ave. near Lincoln Rd., 718-287-3400

**Litchfield Villa** Prospect Park W. and 5th St., 718-965-8900

**Brooklyn Center for the Urban Environment** Tennis House, near Prospect Park W. and 9th St., 718-788-8500

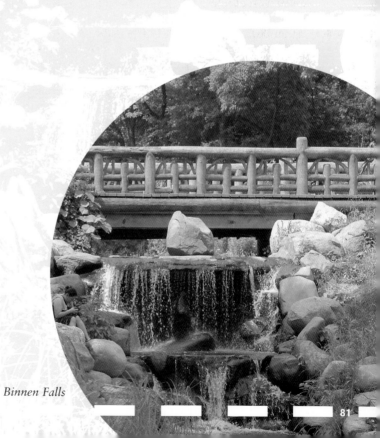

*Binnen Falls*

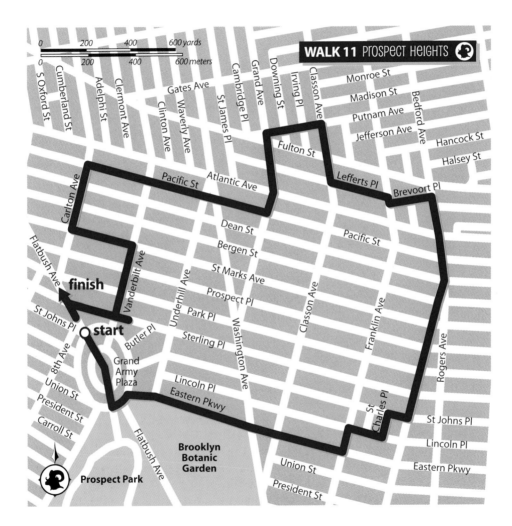

0 200 400 600 yards
0 200 400 600 meters

S Oxford St
Cumberland Pl
Adelphi St
Clermont Ave
Clinton Ave
Waverly Ave
St James Pl
Cambridge Pl
Grand Ave
Downing St
Irving Pl
Classon Ave

Monroe St
Madison St
Putnam Ave
Jefferson Ave
Bedford Ave
Hancock St
Halsey St

Gates Ave

Fulton St

Lefferts Pl
Brevoort Pl

Carlton Ave
Pacific St
Atlantic Ave

Dean St
Pacific St

Bergen St

St Marks Ave

Flatbush Ave
finish

Vanderbilt Ave
Underhill Ave
Prospect Pl
Washington Ave
Classon Ave
Franklin Ave
Rogers Ave

St Johns Pl
Park Pl
Butler Pl
start
Sterling Pl

8th Ave
Union St
President St
Carroll St

Grand
Army
Plaza

Lincoln Pl
Eastern Pkwy

St Charles Pl

St Johns Pl
Lincoln Pl
Eastern Pkwy

Flatbush Ave

Brooklyn
Botanic
Garden

Union St
President St

Prospect Park

# 11 Prospect Heights: Cluster of Cultural Landmarks

BOUNDARIES: **Flatbush Ave., Putnam Ave., Bedford Ave., Eastern Pkwy.**
DISTANCE: **Approx. 3¾ miles**
SUBWAY: **2 or 3 to Grand Army Plaza**

Prospect Heights may be the richest neighborhood in Brooklyn—not in income, but in institutions. The Brooklyn Museum, Brooklyn Public Library, and Brooklyn Botanic Garden are all located here, as well as Grand Army Plaza, which marks the northern entrance to Prospect Park. Promoted with the marketing slogan "Heart of Brooklyn," the area is sometimes referred to as Institute Park, after the museum's original name (Brooklyn Institute of Arts and Sciences). Prospect Heights is also a great comeback story. Its population dropped by more than 25 percent in the 1970s as residents decamped for the suburbs, but since the 1990s, brownstone lovers have been drifting over from Park Slope in pursuit of lower real-estate prices. The population is still heavily West Indian, as it is in neighboring Crown Heights.

- The angel-themed artwork in the subway station is an homage to the angels atop the Grand Army Plaza arch, which you'll soon see. Exit the subway on the north side of Flatbush Ave. and walk toward the traffic circle. With the bust of Alexander J.C. Skene (a Union Army surgeon and later pioneering gynecologist) on your left, cross the street, then immediately cross to your right to approach Bailey Fountain. The man and woman standing in the center represent Wisdom and Felicity. In the water are Tritons and Neptune. Look for the chubby child and his horn of plenty at the man's knee.

- Walk through the stupendous Soldiers' and Sailors' Memorial Arch, passing President Lincoln on your right and General Grant on your left. Their horses were sculpted by painter Thomas Eakins, a good friend of Brooklynite Walt Whitman (whom Eakins painted). Once through the arch, turn around to see the Union army depicted in the sculptural grouping on the left and the navy on the right. Take a few minutes to study these stirring tributes and look for easily missed details. Note the fallen—a soldier lying prone before the angel in the army tableau, a sailor slumped on the left side of the navy group. Frederick MacMonnies, the sculptor, used himself as the model for the army officer brandishing a sword at front. He also included a black man in the navy scene (crouching next to the cannon), making this one of the few Civil War monuments to portray an African-American. The arch is topped by a sculpture formally named *Quadriga,* which refers to the four-horse chariot ridden by Columbia (representing the United States) and two angels of victory.

- With your back to the arch, use the crosswalk on your right, then cross to your left. You'll be at the entrance of Prospect Park, with its four eagle sentries. The statue of James Stranahan, the businessman who spearheaded the park's creation, was sculpted by the same artist who did the arch sculptures and entrance eagles, Frederick MacMonnies.

- Walk alongside the park and cross Flatbush Ave. to the main branch of the Brooklyn Public Library and its brand-new 16,000-square-foot plaza—an outdoor coffeehouse, if you will. The library's prime outside attraction had always been its 40-foot doors, featuring bronze sculptings of literary characters and authors. The two women in the top row are Hester Prynne (left) and *Little Women*'s Meg March. Tom Sawyer is at the bottom left, with Rip Van Winkle two panels above him. The animals include Moby Dick, Edgar Allan Poe's raven, Brer Rabbit, Paul Bunyan's blue ox Babe, and a howling White Fang from the Jack London novel. Walt Whitman is depicted above Wynken, Blynken, and Nod in their wooden-shoe boat. This 1941 building, which is listed on the National Register of Historic Places, resembles an open book when viewed from above. The library is also worth seeing inside, where exhibitions of art, photography, and literature are held.

- Turn right and walk on Eastern Pkwy. Quotations about books and reading are inscribed on all sides of the library, including words from Shakespeare ("Come and take choice . . . ") and Thoreau ("Books are the treasured wealth . . ."), among others.

- Past the library, climb the stairs on your right into Mount Prospect Park, the second-highest point in Brooklyn. It was used as a lookout by the Continental Army during the Revolutionary War and was supposed to be part of Prospect Park. But Frederick Law Olmsted and Calvert Vaux objected to a busy road (part of Flatbush Ave.) running through the bucolic park they were designing. Walk across the lawn or on the path around it; from the far side, you can see the statues atop the Brooklyn Museum. Exit down the path, with the playground on your left.

- Go right on Eastern Pkwy., past an entrance to the Brooklyn Botanic Garden (see page 95), and then you are at the Brooklyn Museum, a Beaux Arts stunner from 1893. The allegorical female sculptures flanking the colonnade were crafted by Daniel Chester French, of Lincoln Memorial fame, to represent Manhattan and (with the boy) Brooklyn. They were created in 1916 for the Brooklyn entrance to the Manhattan Bridge and were moved to the museum when displaced by road reconstruction in 1963. The museum is entered through a glass-encased semicircle protruding from the bottom—a jarring modernist intrusion.

- Continue on Eastern Pkwy., passing the dancing waters that debuted in 2004 with the glass entry pavilion. Cross Washington Ave. and go into Dr. Ronald McNair Park on the right. Proceed to the three-sided obelisk that displays bronze images of *Challenger* astronaut McNair and his accomplishments—including his black belt in karate—and inscriptions of his thoughts on the universe. Beyond it is a granite urn honoring the park's previous namesake, Joseph Guider, who served Brooklyn as an assemblyman, public works commissioner, and borough president.

- Back on Eastern Pkwy., you pass from Prospect Heights into Crown Heights, but Messrs. Olmsted and Vaux would have wanted you to keep walking. They created Eastern Pkwy. and its pedestrian mall as part of their Prospect Park design and as part of a grander plan to link NYC parks with landscaped boulevards and green spaces. That vision was unfulfilled, but

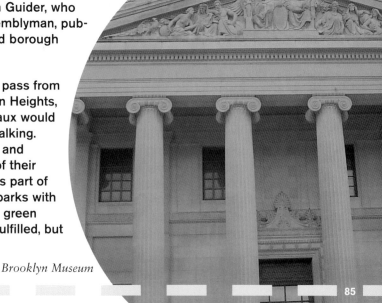

*Brooklyn Museum*

their lovely concept for this, the world's first six-lane parkway, and the similar Ocean Pkwy. that extends south from the park, earned the roads recognition by the National Register of Historic Places.

- Turn left on Franklin Ave., quickly followed by a right on Lincoln Pl. Check out St. Francis Pl. on your left, then turn left on its equally charming sibling, St. Charles Pl.

- Turn right on St. John's Pl. and left on Bedford Ave. The car showroom turned residential building at the next corner still bears the name Studebaker, the automobile manufacturer that ceased production in 1966. At Bergen St., look for faces in the capitals of the Corinthian columns of the slightly forlorn Washington Temple on your left. You'll then approach Ulysses S. Grant, astride his horse between several lanes of vehicular traffic, from behind. The chateaulike apartment house on your right between Dean and Pacific is the Imperial, one of several illustrious buildings nearby. When it was constructed in 1892, apartment living was uncommon for the well-to-do, so the building featured opulent and spacious units to lure them in. You can dip down

## THE BROOKLYN MUSEUM

The Brooklyn Museum is a world-class institution that never loses sight of its local community. At any given time, you'll probably find at least one exhibition showcasing New York artists or themes. On the same visit, you can tour top-notch collections from Africa, Asia, and the Islamic world. The museum may be best known for its Egyptian collection, which includes pieces from 3500 B.C. through A.D. 395. Other highlights are the fully furnished and decorated period rooms, Rodin sculptures, and European paintings (including canvases by Goya, Picasso, and French impressionists). The galleries of American art feature paintings by Cole, Eakins, Sargent, and O'Keeffe, as well as furniture, textiles, and household and decorative objects. A signature holding of the museum is in its American collection—the circa-1820 painting *Winter Scene in Brooklyn* by Francis Guy. In 2007 the museum gave Judy Chicago's *The Dinner Party* a permanent home in its brand-new Elizabeth A. Sackler Center for Feminist Art, which also has galleries for temporary exhibits. An outdoor space is filled with sculpture and other architectural ornamentation salvaged from demolished NYC structures.

Pacific to your right for a look at St. Bartholomew's, a country church built in the city in the late 1880s.

- Back on Bedford Ave., that immense red-brick castle on your left is an armory built around 1892 for the 23rd Regiment of New York's National Guard. Their World War I losses are paid tribute in a bronze tableau on the structure near Atlantic Ave.

- Cross Atlantic Ave. and turn left on Brevoort Pl.—brownstone heaven since the 1860s.

- Turn right on Franklin Ave. and then make a quick left on Lefferts Pl., walking beneath the train trestle. The interesting assortment of homes on this block includes a sideways mansion on the right (probably built before the current streets were laid out) and the contiguous sextet with oriel windows on the left.

- Turn right on Classon Ave., and then go left on Putnam Ave., where a mechanics union has its headquarters in the vertiginous landmark structure built for the Lincoln Club, an organization of Republicans, in 1889. The club's initials interlock on the gable beside the bizarre half tower of this Renaissance/Romanesque melange. Continuing on Putnam, you may want to make a side trip down Downing St., depending on how big a fan you are of the 2006 movie *Dave Chappelle's Block Party,* filmed here.

- Turn left from Putnam onto Grand Ave. Proceed across Fulton St., past an 1885 church (now serving Seventh Day Adventists) that's busy with windows and wings in a multitude of shapes. Turn right on Pacific St., where you'll pass another imposing church, St. Joseph's.

- Turn left on Carlton Ave., central avenue of the Prospect Heights national historic district and emblematic of the beautiful late-Victorian residential architecture that merited that designation. Brownstones rule here, though the exceptions are alluring too, whether it's the extra-tall #575 with private courtyard and sidewalk garden or its sprawling brick neighbor across Bergen St. with a tiled-roof conical tower.

- Turn left on St. Mark's Ave., another gorgeous block, and then go right on Vanderbilt Ave. The buildings on your left after Park Pl. present a nifty arrangement of round, pyramidal, and dormered roofs. Go left on Sterling Pl. for a full view of former P.S. 9, the alma mater of *Appalachian Spring* composer Aaron Copland.

- Turn back and walk west on Sterling Pl. Across Vanderbilt St. is an even older school building, now occupied by P.S. 340. Farther along on the right is the appropriately named Majestic apartment house. It's followed by a series of late-19th-century brownstones that curves around onto Flatbush Ave. Look up to see what's special about this group of buildings.

- Turn left on Flatbush Ave., and you can turn around for an even better view of the Sterling/Flatbush brownstones. On this block of Flatbush, enjoy a taste of the Caribbean at Christie's. Run by the same family for more than 40 years, Christie's doles out tasty meat patties and coco bread—if you order them together, they're served as a sandwich.

- Go back across Sterling Pl. to the B and Q trains' 7th Ave. station at Flatbush Ave. and Park Pl.

## POINTS OF INTEREST

**Brooklyn Public Library** Flatbush Ave. and Eastern Pkwy., Brooklyn, NY 11238, 718-230-2100

**Mount Prospect Park** Eastern Pkwy. at Underhill Ave., Brooklyn, NY 11238

**Brooklyn Museum** 200 Eastern Pkwy., Brooklyn, NY 11238, 718-638-5000

**Dr. Ronald McNair Park** Eastern Pkwy. and Washington Ave., Brooklyn, NY 11225

**Christie's Jamaican Patties** 387 Flatbush Ave., Brooklyn, NY 11238, 718-636-9746

*Soldiers' and Sailors' Memorial Arch*

# route summary

1. Begin at Grand Army Plaza.
2. Cross over to the Prospect Park entrance.
3. Cross Flatbush Ave. to the Brooklyn Public Library and turn right on Eastern Pkwy.
4. Turn left on Franklin Ave. and right on Lincoln Pl.
5. Turn left on St. Charles Pl.
6. Turn right on St. John's Pl.
7. Turn left on Bedford Ave.
8. Cross Atlantic Ave. and turn left on Brevoort Pl.
9. Turn right on Franklin and make a quick left on Lefferts Pl.
10. Turn right on Classon Ave., then left on Putnam Ave.
11. Turn left on Grand Ave., then right on Pacific St.
12. Turn left on Carlton Ave.
13. Turn left on St. Mark's Ave., then right on Vanderbilt Ave.
14. Go left on Sterling Pl., then turn back and walk west on Sterling.
15. Turn left on Flatbush Ave.
16. Turn around and walk north on Flatbush to Park Pl. for the subway.

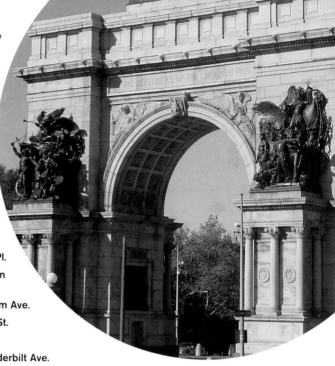

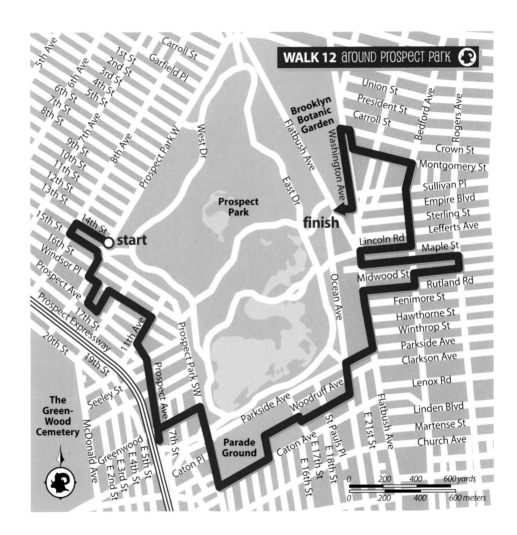

WALK 12 around Prospect Park

Brooklyn Botanic Garden

Prospect Park

The Green-Wood Cemetery

Parade Ground

start

finish

5th Ave
6th Ave
7th Ave
8th Ave
Carroll St
Garfield Pl
1st St
2nd St
3rd St
4th St
5th St
6th St
7th St
8th St
9th St
10th St
11th St
12th St
13th St
15th St
14th St
16th St
Windsor Pl
Prospect Ave
17th St
20th St
19th St
Prospect Expressway
Seeley St
McDonald Ave
Greenwood
E 5th St
E 4th St
E 3rd St
E 2nd St
7th St
Caton Pl
Caton Ave
Prospect Ave
Prospect Park SW
11th Ave
Prospect Park W
West Dr
8th Ave
7th Ave
East Dr
Flatbush Ave
Washington Ave
Union St
President St
Carroll St
Bedford Ave
Rogers Ave
Crown St
Montgomery St
Sullivan Pl
Empire Blvd
Sterling St
Lefferts Ave
Lincoln Rd
Maple St
Midwood St
Rutland Rd
Fenimore St
Hawthorne St
Winthrop St
Parkside Ave
Clarkson Ave
Lenox Rd
Linden Blvd
Martense St
Church Ave
Ocean Ave
Parkside Ave
Woodruff Ave
St Pauls Pl
E 17th St
E 18th St
E 16th St
E 21st St
Flatbush Ave

0   200   400   600 yards
0   200   400   600 meters

# 12 around prospect park: skirting the perimeter

**BOUNDARIES:** 8th Ave., 18th St., Caton Ave., Rogers Ave., Montgomery St.
**DISTANCE:** Approx. 5¼ miles
**SUBWAY:** F to 15th St.

This is a lengthy walk from the westernmost to easternmost point of Prospect Park. It's no straight line, and you never set foot inside the park. Instead, the walk skirts the park, taking you through Windsor Terrace south to the Parade Ground and then north through Prospect Lefferts Gardens to the Botanic Garden. One of the last stops is the most hallowed place in this "city of churches"—the site of Ebbets Field. It has been an apartment complex for more than 40 years but still exerts an emotional pull on baseball fans, Brooklyn nostalgists, and, perhaps, on anyone who has ever had his or her heart broken.

- After exiting through the subway turnstile, look for the PARK WEST sign in tile on the wall next to a Metrocard machine. Follow that arrow, going up the first staircase on your right after it. You'll be facing the Pavilion multiplex, which predates the multiplex era, originating in 1926 as a single-screen cinema.

- Walk west—away from Prospect Park—on 14th St. Some call this area South Slope, as opposed to Park Slope on the other side of 10th St. But this block is pure Park Slope in style, from the elegant Montauk apartment house on the right corner to the plethora of brownstones and brickfronts.

- At 8th Ave., glimpse stately P.S. 107 to your right, but turn left and take in the fortresslike 14th Regiment Armory. It was erected in 1895, a year after the school, and contains a stone from the Gettysburg battlefield to the right of the front door.

- Turn left on 15th St. and proceed into Bartel-Pritchard Square, a circle centered on a black granite war memorial. Bartel and Pritchard were two Brooklyn boys killed in World War I. Opposite, two columns designed by Stanford White gird the entrance to Prospect Park. The leafy embellishment on the columns was copied from the Acanthus Column of Delphi, named for the acanthus plant whose leaves are represented in it.

- Walk away from the park on Prospect Park W. You are now in Windsor Terrace, home to many police officers and firefighters. Windsor Terrace native Vincent E. Brunton, for whom 16th St. is now named, was a fire department captain who died in the World Trade Center collapse. He moonlighted as a bartender at Farrell's, the old-time saloon on your left at 16th that's said to be one of the first bars opened in Brooklyn after Prohibition was repealed. Cops, firefighters, and neighborhood loyalists love Farrell's, which was featured in a scene with Helen Hunt and Shirley Knight in the Oscar-winning flick *As Good As It Gets.* The Western Union outlet across 16th was Harvey Keitel's shop in *Smoke. Dog Day Afternoon* was filmed a few blocks farther on Prospect Park W., between 17th and 18th Sts. You can walk down to see the bank Al Pacino robs, though it's now unrecognizable, having been converted from a warehouse into condos.

- From Farrell's, proceed south on Prospect Park W. and turn left on Windsor Pl. Turn right on Howard Pl., left on Prospect Ave., and left on Fuller Pl. The rowhouses on Howard and Fuller don't have the same pedigree as Park Slope's, but they're attractive nonetheless.

- Turn right on Windsor Pl. and take it to 11th Ave., where you turn right. Go left on Prospect Ave. Immediately past Greenwood Ave. on your left is a firehouse constructed in 1896 of brick, limestone, and slate. It was originally manned by volunteers, who watched for fires from the tower that's now boarded up.

- Turn around and go right on Greenwood Ave. Cross E. 7th, also named for a firefighter (Jeff Palazzo) killed on 9/11. Continue to Prospect Park S.W., cross to the park side, and turn right. Walk around a colonnaded pavilion—created, believe it or not, for public transit passengers. This pair of shelters (another one is across the road) were designed by Stanford White in 1896. A few years later, the dramatic *Horse Tamers* sculptures flanking this entrance to the park were unveiled. The artist was Frederick MacMonnies, who did several pieces for the park.

- Cross Parkside Ave., then go left on Caton Ave. Enter the Parade Ground through the arch on your left. This space was established at the same time as Prospect Park, solely for staging military pageants. It has, of course, provided many more years of service for athletics than for military events, starting with cricket, archery, and lawn bowling. When Brooklyn caught baseball fever in the late 19th century, 20 fields were added, and the Parade Ground has been *the* place for amateur baseball ever since. Sandy Koufax, Joe Torre, Willie Randolph, and Manny Ramirez were all scouted by the pros while playing here.

● Turn right at the concession kiosk and exit onto Parade Pl., right in front of the regal Warlyn apartments. Go to your right, then go left on Crooke Ave. Here's an oddity at #20 on your right: was a modern high-rise built on top of a Dutch Colonial house, or a Dutch Colonial front faked for a modern high-rise? Farther along, Holbrook Hall at #36 is one small example of British names being adopted for prestige, a tactic favored by early residential developers around Prospect Park's southern end. Continue past St. Paul's Pl. and a series of detached houses on your right.

● Turn left on Ocean Ave., one of Brooklyn's grand boulevards, known for its classic apartment buildings. Examine and admire the detail on #365, #361, #353, and #354.

● At Parkside Ave., you've reached another entrance to Prospect Park. No statues at this southeast tip, just a pergola—the shelter of granite columns. Go right and check out Parkside Ct. on your left on your way to Flatbush Ave.

● Turn left on Flatbush, first taking note of the whimsical rooflines diagonally across the intersection, with their peekaboo apertures and sphere-on-pedestal sculptings. Glance down a few more cul-de-sacs to the left off Flatbush—first Westbury Ct., where some apartment houses have elaborate ornamentation, then Chester Ct., whose tidy rowhouses combine Tudor fronts with Spanish-tile roofs. These

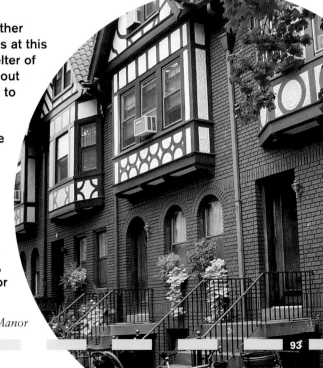

*Rutland Rd. in Lefferts Manor*

are your first samplings of the fine turn-of-the-century residences and varied architectural styles here in Prospect Lefferts Gardens.

● Turn right on Rutland Rd.—astoundingly peaceful compared to bustling Flatbush Ave.
that you just left. You're now within the bounds of Lefferts Manor, the original development that grew into Prospect Lefferts Gardens. While outsiders might consider the
whole area part of Flatbush, those who live in "the Manor" keep the distinctions alive.
In the 1890s, with the new Prospect Park an attractive local amenity and the even
newer Brooklyn Bridge easing the commute to Manhattan, communities were developed around Flatbush. This one was initiated by a member of the Lefferts family, who
had been farming this land since 1660. He divided his property into 600 lots and sold
them on the condition that each buyer build only a single-family home, made of brick
or stone, set back from the street at least 14 feet. Construction continued into the
1920s.

● Turn left on Bedford Ave. and right on Midwood St. Then go left on Rogers Ave. and
left on Maple St., a street nicknamed Doctors Row after the profession still common
to several of its residents.

● When you reach Flatbush, you can dine in or take out from Mike's International across
the avenue. They make patties, roti, tropical drinks, and other West Indian specialties. Then walk north on Flatbush, and turn right on Lincoln Rd. The frame houses
on the right appear to violate the original restrictions on home construction in the
area, though they were built in the first wave of development. An older structure, the
terra cotta and brick Grace Reformed Church (1893), is on your left at the corner with
Bedford Ave.

● Turn left on Bedford Ave. Look down charming Lefferts Ave. and Sterling St. as you
pass them. At Empire Blvd., you cross into Crown Heights. Proceed toward the massive and foreboding high-rises at Sullivan Pl. This is what's become of Ebbets Field,
ballpark of the Brooklyn Dodgers—a team that captured the hearts and minds of fans
like no other team in any sport, that put an end to the ban on black players, that made
up for years of agony with one World Series victory over the Yankees, and that two
years later was packed up and taken to Los Angeles by owner Walter O'Malley, who
would be reviled in Brooklyn for generations. "Dem Bums" played their final innings

on these acres in September 1957, and their stadium was razed in 1960. Somewhere, someone is weeping about it today.

- Turn left on Montgomery St. Medgar Evers College is on your right; an elementary school named for the Dodgers' civil rights icon, Jackie Robinson, is on McKeever Pl. to your left. Past McKeever, a cute playground offers dancing polar bears that spray water in the summer. Then the street turns dingy—industrialized and graffitied.

- Turn right on Washington Ave. The walk concludes at the Brooklyn Botanic Garden. Its Japanese garden, featuring a pond, wooden bridges, and Shinto shrine, is many New Yorkers' favorite place to escape the frenetic urban pace. The Botanic Garden also contains Brooklyn's version of the Hollywood Walk of Fame—a path of stones inscribed with names of famous Brooklynites. About 13,000 plant species are found within the garden's 52 acres.

- From the Botanic Garden gate, walk south on Washington and turn right on Empire Blvd. to get the B or Q train at Flatbush Ave.

## POINTS OF INTEREST

**Farrell's** 215 Prospect Park W., Brooklyn, NY 11215, 718-788-8779

**Parade Ground** Parkside to Caton Ave. at Coney Island Ave., Brooklyn, NY 11218, 718-438-3435

**Mike's International** 552 Flatbush Ave., Brooklyn, NY 11225, 718-856-7034

**Brooklyn Botanic Garden** 1000 Washington Ave., Brooklyn, NY 11225, 718-623-7200

## route summary

1. From Prospect Park W., walk west on 14th St.
2. Turn left on 8th Ave.
3. Turn left on 15th St.
4. Cross Bartel-Pritchard Square to Prospect Park W. and head south.
5. Turn left on Windsor Pl., right on Howard Pl., left on Prospect Ave., and left on Fuller Pl.
6. Go right on Windsor, right on 11th Ave., and left on Prospect past Greenwood Ave.
7. Turn around and go right on Greenwood Ave.
8. Turn right on Prospect Park S.W.
9. Cross Parkside Ave. and turn left on Caton Ave.
10. Enter the Parade Ground from Caton; exit on Parade Pl. and go right.
11. Turn left on Crooke Ave.
12. Go left on Ocean Ave.
13. Turn right on Parkside Ave.
14. Turn left on Flatbush Ave.
15. Go right on Rutland Rd.
16. Turn left on Bedford Ave., right on Midwood St., left on Rogers Ave., and left on Maple St.
17. Go right on Flatbush, followed by a right on Lincoln Rd.
18. Turn left on Bedford.
19. Go left on Montgomery St.
20. Turn right on Washington Ave. for the Brooklyn Botanic Garden.
21. Walk south on Washington to Empire Blvd., then turn right and proceed to the Prospect Park subway station at Flatbush.

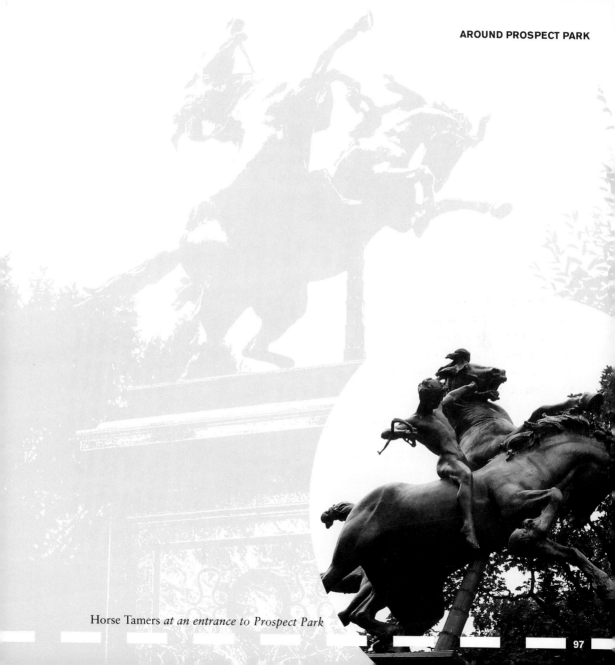

Horse Tamers *at an entrance to Prospect Park*

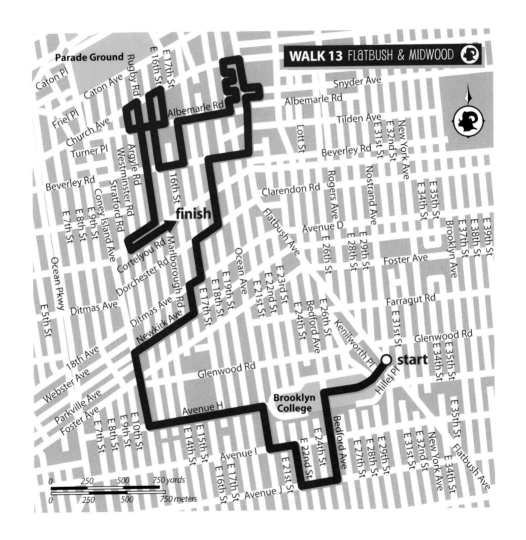

WALK 13 FLATBUSH & MIDWOOD

Parade Ground

Caton Pl
Caton Ave
Friel Pl
Church Ave
Turner Pl
Beverley Rd
Rugby Rd
E 17th St
E 16th St
Albemarle Rd
Argyle Rd
Westminster Rd
Stratford Rd
Coney Island Ave
E 9th St
E 8th St
E 7th St
16th St
Ocean Pkwy
E 5th St
Ditmas Ave
18th Ave
Webster Ave
Parkville Ave
Foster Ave
E 7th St
E 8th St
E 9th St
E 10th St
E 15th St
E 14th St
E 17th St
E 16th St
Cortelyou Rd
Marlborough Rd
Dorchester Rd
Ditmas Ave
Newkirk Ave
finish
Glenwood Rd
Avenue H
Avenue I
Avenue J

Snyder Ave
Albemarle Rd
Tilden Ave
Lott St
Beverley Rd
Clarendon Rd
Avenue D
Flatbush Ave
Ocean Ave
E 19th St
E 18th St
E 17th St
E 23rd St
E 22nd St
E 21st St
E 26th St
Bedford Ave
E 24th St
Rogers Ave
Nostrand Ave
E 26th St
E 29th St
E 28th St
Foster Ave
Farragut Rd
Kenilworth Pl
E 31st St
Glenwood Rd
E 21st St
E 22nd St
E 24th St
Bedford Ave
E 27th St
E 28th St
E 29th St
E 31st St
E 32nd St
New York Ave
Flatbush Ave

E 32nd St
E 31st St
New York Ave
E 34th St
E 35th St
E 38th St
E 37th St
E 39th St
Brooklyn Ave
E 34th St
E 35th St

start
Hillel Pl

Brooklyn
College

0   250   500   750 yards
0   250   500   750 meters

98

# 13 FLATBUSH AND MIDWOOD: SUBURBAN SPLENDOR IN THE HEART OF THE CITY

**BOUNDARIES: Nostrand Ave., Avenue J, Coney Island Ave., Church Ave.**
**DISTANCE: Approx. 5½ miles**
**SUBWAY: 2 or 5 to Flatbush Ave./Brooklyn College**

Only a few neighborhood names are instantly recognized by nonresidents. The Left Bank is one. The French Quarter another. In Brooklyn, Flatbush has earned that honor. Non–New Yorkers got to know Flatbush from the movies, the Dodgers (who actually played in Crown Heights), and from local boys and girls made good (there are a lot of them!). Virtually all the black-and-white images and clichés about "growing up in Brooklyn" sprang from the streets of Flatbush, as did the writers, filmmakers, and sentimentalists who spread them around the world. This walk groups Flatbush with Midwood, just as Dutch settlers did in the 1650s when they called the whole area both Midwout and Vlackebos (both names refer to woods). Midwood today is largely identified with its Orthodox Jewish population, though it's also where you'll find one of New York's top-rated pizzerias (DiFara at Avenue J and E. 15th) and a strip known as Little Pakistan. Flatbush, once a stronghold of Jewish immigrant families, is home to many West Indians and a jumble of other ethnicities. It also includes about a dozen mini-neighborhoods developed as posh suburban communities at the turn of the century and now known collectively as Victorian Flatbush. The glorious homes here—not all of them strictly Victorian in style—are a hidden gem of residential Brooklyn.

● From the busy intersection where you emerge from the subway, walk on Hillel Pl. to Brooklyn College. This public university held its first classes in Downtown Brooklyn in the late 1920s. This campus was built in 1937 with $5 million in New Deal funds. Upon entering the campus, you'll see the sculpture *Survival,* a powerful depiction of those who had to rebuild their lives after the Holocaust. The school's performing arts center, which books well-known artists, is to your left. Go to your right, then turn left on the path between Boylan and Whitehead halls and proceed to the college's emblematic structure, its Georgian-style library. Go down the stairs in front of the library and step onto the quad. Brooklyn College had a reputation for liberalism well before the 1960s student protests that took place on this green. The college was derisively called "the little red schoolhouse" even before the House Un-American Activities Committee subpoenaed several professors and the student government and newspaper were suspended over alleged communist sympathies in the 1950s. Administrators have always preferred the school's other nickname anyway: "the poor man's Harvard." Alumni include novelist Irwin Shaw, film director Paul Mazursky, attorney Alan Dershowitz, U.S. senator Barbara Boxer, author Frank McCourt, actor Jimmy Smits, and numerous other boldface names.

● Exit the campus on the far side of the green, at Bedford Ave., and go left on Bedford. Roosevelt Hall on your right, the school's original gym, was renamed for FDR in 1947. The president had laid its cornerstone back in 1936, proud to support an institution that served the nonwealthy and provided employment during the Depression for construction workers.

● Turn right on Avenue J, then turn right on E. 22nd St. The sideways house on your right at #1041 is a city landmark, one of the dozen or so Dutch farmhouses still standing in Brooklyn. Known as the Johannes Van Nuyse (or Van Nuyse-Magaw) House, it was built at what's now 22nd and M in 1803 and moved here in 1916. It had to be placed perpendicular to the street to fit the lot. The entrance portico on the left side was added in 1952.

● Turn left on Avenue I, right on Ocean Ave., and left on Avenue H. The century-old subway station at E. 16th St., which resembles a rural train depot, is one of the city's last such structures made of wood. It had been slated for demolition, due to fire safety concerns, but was granted landmark status. Continue on H.

● Turn right at Coney Island Ave. for a brief tour of Little Pakistan. The Makki Mosque and community center on your right are lifelines of this community, which was drastically affected by 9/11. At least 30 businesses closed and up to half the residents left or were deported after the government started requiring registration of immigrants from Muslim countries. Pak Sweets & Grill, on your left at Parkville Ave., offers all kinds of homemade Pakistani pastries, candy, and hot food.

● Turn right on Newkirk Ave. beside elegant P.S. 217. On your right after Rugby Rd., the B and Q subway tracks are sunken from street level in what's known as an open cut, which residents preferred to an elevated train when the city decided to eliminate all street-level rail lines around 1907.

- Turn left on E. 16th, the central north-south artery of Ditmas Park, a part of Victorian Flatbush designated as a national historic district. It was created by developer Lewis Pounds in 1902. The streets and sidewalks were paved, sewers installed, and land-scaping done before any houses were built. Another stricture set by Pounds: no two homes could be identical. There are two interlopers on your left at #578 and #574, built in the 1880s and later transported to these lots. The rest of the block dates to 1909 and consists of mostly California bungalow–style homes designed by Pounds's preferred architect, Arlington Isham.

- Turn right on Ditmas Ave., the middle east-west avenue of the historic district. Mary Pickford and Douglas Fairbanks, the Brangelina of their time, lived on Ditmas when they were making movies at Vitagraph, a top film studio prior to 1920. Vitagraph eventually relocated from Midwood to Hollywood and was bought by Warner Bros. The property, at E. 14th St. near Avenue M, was used into the 1980s for TV produc-tions like Steve Allen's and Perry Como's variety hours and *The Cosby Show.*

- Turn left on E. 17th St. The classic Victorian at #484 is an Isham design from 1902.

- Turn right at Dorchester Rd. On your right between 18th and 19th Sts. stands the Flatbush Tompkins Congregational Church, erected in 1910. The parish house behind the church on 18th has a completely dif-ferent look: shingled, with dissimilar doors on either end of its multisided bulge and topped by a pyramidal roof with tall dormer windows.

*A house in Victorian Flatbush*

- From Dorchester, turn left on E. 19th St. The house at #257 was visited by Denzel Washington, playing the title role, in the Spike Lee film *Malcolm X*. The one at #247 might be described as a confused plantation home. A pastel green color is just one of the unusual features of the manse at #235.

- Go right on Beverley Rd. At Ocean Ave., known for its handsome apartment houses, look for the sculptures above the first-floor windows on the corner building on your left. Is this old man exhausted or perplexed? A scholar or an artist? In the Vitagraph studio's heyday, this building was home to many movie stars.

- Proceed on Beverley to Flatbush Ave. and go left. The Loews Kings on your right was Flatbush's grandest movie palace and a center of neighborhood social life from its opening in 1929 until TV started changing viewing habits. You didn't come to the Kings just to see a *pickchuh;* you'd see a double feature plus a newsreel, travelogue, and cartoons. A teenage Barbra Streisand worked as an usher here. After the 3,000-seat theater closed in 1977, the city bought it to prevent its demolition.

- Turn right at Snyder Ave. to visit a relic from another bygone era. As an independent municipality, Flatbush built this quaint town hall on your left in 1875. Two decades later, Flatbush was annexed by the city of Brooklyn, disempowering its seat of government.

- Go back to Flatbush and turn right. You may have heard of Erasmus Hall as the high school where Barbra Streisand and Neil Diamond were classmates, or as the alma mater of many other famous people, but that advance hype probably doesn't prepare you for the gargantuan neo-Gothic edifice on your right. Erasmus Hall was chartered as a public school in 1895, and before this building was erected in 1903 it occupied a Georgian-Federal schoolhouse built by the private Erasmus Hall Academy in 1787. That original school, porch and all, still stands in the courtyard. Erasmus Hall Academy was the second school founded in the United States, and it was organized by the Flatbush Reformed Dutch Church across the avenue. This was one of Brooklyn's three original Reformed churches, established in the mid-17th century by Peter Stuyvesant, who headed the Dutch colony/city of New Amsterdam.

- Turn left on Church Ave. and then go left on E. 21st St. into another of Victorian Flatbush's national historic districts. This one is composed of just the two cul-de-sacs to your left, Kenmore Terr. and Albemarle Terr. Go in and out of both. The church's 1853 parsonage is the only detached house on Kenmore, which was developed in 1918 with such suburban amenities as driveways and lawns. Albemarle, built two years earlier, is lined with Federal-style brick rowhouses.

● Turn right from E. 21st onto Albemarle Rd., in front of the Salem Missionary Baptist Church. This African-American congregation, which has moved into a former synagogue, was founded in 1910 for the servants who worked in the mansions of Prospect Park South and environs.

● Turn left on E. 17th St. and go right on Beverley. The 100-year-old subway station on your left at E. 16th was spruced up in the 1990s with an artwork called *Garden Stops,* comprising the hand-etched windows and wrought-iron railings with floral patterns.

● Turn right at Marlborough Rd., one of the British names that replaced numbered streets when Dean Alvord created Prospect Park South, the swankiest development carved out of the town of Flatbush at the turn of the century. Alvord envisioned a garden enclave within the city and included such features as landscaped medians. For an even greater air of exclusivity, Alvord installed gateposts engraved with "PPS" along Beverley (or Beverly, as it's spelled on these brick structures), which still flank each side street. Note the "CS" on the chimney of 187 Marlborough Rd. on your right. Charles Stillwell, who had the house built, was a descendant of the Stillwell family, early English settlers in Gravesend for whom Coney Island's Stillwell Ave. was named. Intrepid reporter Nellie Bly lived for a while in the house opposite at #184.

● Turn right at Church Ave., passing Temple Beth Emeth on your right. The Little Jewel Box, as this 1913 synagogue has been nicknamed, has its original stained glass, a marble pulpit, and a bronze arc to hold the Torah. A thousand families belonged to the congregation in the 1930s and '40s; at present, about 120 families worship here.

● Turn right on Buckingham Rd., one of the most extraordinary city streets you're likely to see. It even has its own village green. The mansion with a silo, #115, was home to Gillette of razor fame. The most celebrated mansion is the pagoda-ish #131, known as the Japanese House. Orientalism was in vogue among the upper class of the late 19th century, but usually just one room in a house was decorated in the style. Built as a model house for the community, this house proved to be a tough sell—selling at a loss after three years on the market to a physician who moved out within two years.

- Turn right on Albemarle Rd. Dean Alvord's own home, which later burned down, was located in what's now a woodsy lot across Albemarle. On the right of the gate to the lot are steps from the original house. Many of the Albemarle mansions were built for industry bigwigs of the day, including the chief executives of Fruit of the Loom, Sperry-Rand (progenitor of Unisys), Ex-Lax, and the *Brooklyn Eagle* newspaper.

- Go right on Argyle Rd., right on Church Ave., and then right on Rugby Rd. On your right, Spanish Mission–style #94 is followed by a pseudo-Swiss chalet at #100. Opposite them, #101 is more renowned as the boardinghouse where Meryl Streep lived in *Sophie's Choice.* It was painted pink for filming. When you cross Beverley, you've entered Beverley Square, one of the earliest suburban developments in Flatbush, started in 1898. Residents are trying to gain landmark status for the neighborhood to preserve its integrity, but some say it has already been altered too much. Houses of note on Rugby include #305, called the Honeymoon Cottage because it was built as a wedding present for a Guggenheim daughter; #312, where Brooklyn-born songwriter Arthur Schwartz lived before moving to Hollywood and composing the music for such standards as "Dancing in the Dark" and "That's Entertainment"; and #319, #323, and #324 for their sheer splendidness.

- At Cortelyou Rd., turn right. Look on your right in the yard of 364 Argyle Rd. for the area's last remaining cast-iron street sign. On your left past Westminster Rd., conclude the walk with a meal at the Farm on Adderley. This rustically elegant restaurant uses a variety of fresh, seasonal ingredients in their imaginative soups, appetizers, and entrees. If you just want a snack, try the french fries with curry mayo. Catch the Q train four blocks east at Marlborough.

## POINTS OF INTEREST

**Brooklyn College** 2900 Bedford Ave., Brooklyn, NY 11210, 718-951-5000

**Johannes Van Nuyse House** 1041 E. 22nd St., Brooklyn, NY 11210

**Pak Sweets & Grill** 998 Coney Island Ave., Brooklyn, NY 11230, 718-421-0505

**Erasmus Hall Academy** 911 Flatbush Ave., Brooklyn, NY 11226, 718-282-7804

**The Farm on Adderley** 1108 Cortelyou Rd., Brooklyn, NY 11218, 718-287-3101

## route summary

1. Take Hillel Pl. from Nostrand Ave. to Brooklyn College.
2. Leave the campus on Bedford Ave. and turn left.
3. Turn right on Avenue J, then right on E. 22nd St.
4. Turn left on Avenue I, right on Ocean Ave., and left on Avenue H.
5. Turn right on Coney Island Ave.
6. Turn right on Newkirk Ave.
7. Turn left on E. 16th St.
8. Turn right on Ditmas Ave.
9. Turn left on E. 17th St.
10. Turn right on Dorchester Rd.
11. Turn left on E. 19th St.
12. Turn right on Beverley Rd.
13. Turn left on Flatbush Ave.
14. Go to the right on Snyder Ave., then return to Flatbush and turn right.
15. Go left from Flatbush onto Church Ave., then left again on E. 21st St.
16. Go in and out of both Kenmore and Albemarle Terrs.
17. From E. 21st, turn right at Albemarle Rd.
18. Turn left on E. 17th and right on Beverley.
19. Go right on Marlborough Rd.
20. Turn right on Church.
21. Go right on Buckingham Rd.
22. Turn right on Albemarle Rd.
23. Turn right on Argyle Rd., right on Church, and right on Rugby Rd.
24. Go right on Cortelyou Rd. past Westminster Rd.
25. Turn around and walk east to Marlborough for the Cortelyou Rd. subway.

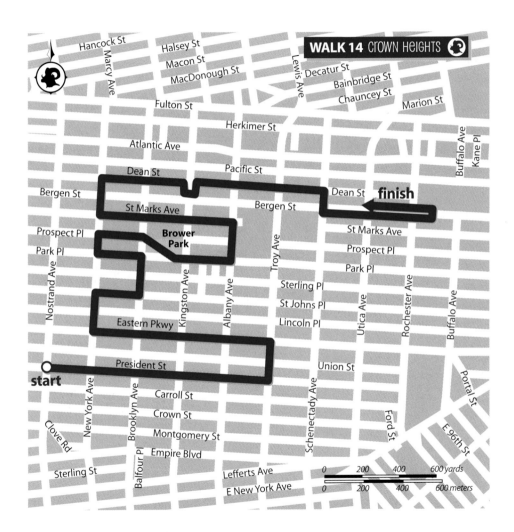

Hancock St
Marcy Ave
Halsey St
Macon St
MacDonough St
Lewis Ave
Decatur St
Bainbridge St
Chauncey St
Marion St
Fulton St
Herkimer St
Buffalo Ave
Kane Pl
Atlantic Ave
Dean St
Pacific St
Bergen St
St Marks Ave
Dean St
**finish**
Bergen St
**Brower Park**
St Marks Ave
Prospect Pl
Prospect Pl
Park Pl
Park Pl
Nostrand Ave
Kingston Ave
Albany Ave
Troy Ave
Sterling Pl
St Johns Pl
Lincoln Pl
Utica Ave
Rochester Ave
Buffalo Ave
Eastern Pkwy
President St
Union St
**start**
New York Ave
Brooklyn Ave
Balfour Pl
Carroll St
Crown St
Montgomery St
Empire Blvd
Schenectady Ave
Ford St
Portal St
E 96th St
Clove Rd
Sterling St
Lefferts Ave
E New York Ave

0    200    400    600 yards
0    200    400    600 meters

# 14 CrOWN HeiGHTS: FINDING COMMON GrOUND

BOUNDARIES: **Nostrand Ave., President St., Buffalo Ave., Dean St.**
DISTANCE: **Approx. 4¼ miles**
SUBWAY: **2 or 5 to President St.**

Crown Heights. It's one of those places, like Selma or Kent State, forever linked in people's minds with a violent event. For Crown Heights, it was three days of rioting in August 1991 that ensued when a seven-year-old black child was fatally struck by a car in the motorcade of Rabbi Menachem Schneerson. A rabbinical student was stabbed to death by black men in retaliation. But Crown Heights has too long a history to be identified with only one incident, and it has a racial heritage to be proud of. In the first generation after slavery, many blacks made their home within the bounds of present-day Crown Heights, establishing towns with schools, churches, and social services. In the 20th century, blacks in Crown Heights introduced a jubilant annual celebration to New York City: the West Indian American Day Parade that attracts more than a million revelers. While tensions remain, the large Caribbean population of Crown Heights has been coexisting peacefully for the last two decades (and the three or four before the riots) with Hasidic Jews of the Lubavitch sect, who have their world head-quarters on Eastern Pkwy. All the hullabaloo over Crown Heights' racial diversity and occa-sional strife has also drawn attention away from its architectural riches. Crown Heights was a wealthy suburb around the turn of the century, and its brownstones, mansions, and churches from those days are as impressive as any in the borough.

● From the subway at Nostrand Ave., walk east on President St. and take in block after block of stunning homes, built mostly during the first three decades of the 20th cen-tury. After you pass Kingston Ave., mansions give way to rowhouses, nonetheless elegant and nicely maintained.

● Turn left on Troy Ave. and go left on Eastern Pkwy. Frederick Law Olmsted invented the word "parkway" for this thoroughfare. He wanted it and Ocean Pkwy., the other Brooklyn parkway he created, to link Prospect Park and Central Park (both of which he codesigned)—thus making nature an integral and continuous presence in the city. Though the plan was never realized, Eastern Pkwy. is a main street of Crown Heights and is pleasant for strolling, with attractive residences within this segment. The

Lubavitchers are concentrated here and to the south, where you just came from. They run the Jewish Children's Museum at the corner of Kingston Ave., where children of all faiths (and ages) are invited to learn about Jewish customs and history. Eastern Pkwy. is also the route of the West Indian American Day Parade. Want to taste the cuisines of Crown Heights? There's a kosher deli inside the museum, or go right one block on Kingston to K&B Carib Kitchen.

- Turn right from Eastern Pkwy. onto New York Ave., which features tall and varied row-houses and some dormers with flourish. Then turn right on St. John's Pl., where there is more uniformity—brownstones on the left, brickfronts on the right.

- Turn left at Brooklyn Ave., a corner commanded by St. Gregory's Catholic Church. This 1915 interpretation of ancient Roman churches was designed by the same architects responsible for the Prospect Park Boathouse, the Williamsburg Trust Company, and the Green Point Savings Bank—all standouts.

- Turn left on Park Pl. A Victorian fortress extends along virtually the entire left side of the block. Regal or foreboding? You decide. It certainly seems too grand to be called a poorhouse, though it was constructed for that purpose by a church in 1889.

- Turn right at New York Ave. Because Crown Heights suffered badly from postwar urban decay, there are a lot of empty old homes in the neighborhood awaiting saviors, i.e., real-estate investors. One example was #196, "The Mansion," on your left across from Trinity Baptist Church. The person who bought it a few years ago did a complete renovation, adding rental apartments on the upper floors and investigating the house's history. He learned that one former occupant was the League School, a pioneer in educating autistic children.

- Turn right on Prospect Pl. and proceed into child-friendly Brower Park, which contains both an elementary school and the Brooklyn Children's Museum. Founded in 1899, it is one of the cultural products of Crown Heights' gilded age (along with the Brooklyn Museum and Brooklyn Botanic Garden). It was the first museum in the world with exhibits on a child-size scale tailored to child interests, and it created the "hands-on" concept. The museum is due to complete a $43 million expansion in late 2007.

● Exit across the park from the school and go left on Park Pl. The Greek temple–style First Church of God in Christ on your right was built as a synagogue in the 1920s. Check out the tiny but classy streets Hampton Pl. and Virginia Pl. to your right, then make a left on Albany Ave.

● Turn left on St. Mark's Ave. So prestigious was this address in the late 1890s, the whole area was called St. Mark's—and immediately recognized as a status symbol. Many of the millionaires' homes have been torn down, but enough remain to keep it a desirable address today. This enviably unique block west of Albany has a playground in the middle of the street and no curbside parking. The double house at #855–#857, with its corner cupola, was designed in 1892 by Montrose Morris, architect of several auspicious residences in nearby Bedford-Stuyvesant. A few doors down, opposite the Children's Museum, the imposing villa at the corner was designed in 1869 by a 33-year-old City College graduate named Russell Sturgis, who would gain renown as an art and architecture critic. Be sure to see its pointed tower with arched windows on Brooklyn Ave.

● Go right on New York Ave. Union United Methodist Church, on your right past Bergen, is a Romanesque classic of red brick and sandstone from 1892. The Hebron church across from it, built in 1909 for the First Church of Christ, Scientist, now serves Seventh Day Adventists of Haitian descent. This intriguing geometry primer features an octagonal sanctuary pierced with triangular gables above long arched windows.

● Turn right on Dean, another nifty street. More ornate dwellings are on the right; the most distinctive on the block are to your left at #1307–#1313. At the Brooklyn Ave. corner on your left, a 50-room mansion

*A Montrose Morris design on St. Mark's Ave.*

was constructed in 1887 for businessman/philanthropist John Truslow by the Parfitt Brothers, preeminent architects of the time. It was eventually subdivided into apartments, declared a city landmark, then embroiled in controversy for over a decade. Its owner was evicted in early 2006 due to unpaid taxes she claimed were improperly assessed. She was judged an unethical landlord by some, a victim of greedy real-estate interests by others. Continuing along Dean, you come to a newly minted landmark: the Elkins House, on your left at #1375. Built sometime between 1854 and 1869, it's the only freestanding wood farmhouse left in this section of Crown Heights.

● Dip down Kingston to your right to refresh with a freshly blended beverage from Heru's Juice Bar. Resume walking east on Dean St. To your right at Albany Ave. is the Paul Robeson School for Business and Technology. A Wall St. brokerage firm offers internships to the school's students, provides tutors, and funds college visits and scholarships—a beneficial partnership no doubt, but somewhat ironic in a school named for a communist. Residences around here include the Weeksville Gardens public housing complex at Troy. Weeksville was a black community established by a longshoreman named James Weeks after slavery was abolished in New York State in 1827. The oft-repeated description of Weeksville as a settlement of freed blacks is inaccurate: not all the people who lived here had been slaves, and quite a few were professionals, including the first black woman doctor in New York State (Susan McKinney Stewart) and the first black Brooklyn police officer (Moses Cobb). The community thrived for nearly a century, with about 300 residents at its peak, and included a nursing home, orphanage, and Colored School No. 2—on the grounds of the current namesake school at Troy. Bethel Tabernacle AME Church, on your right at the Dean/Schenectady corner, was one of Weeksville's churches, founded in 1847. In the 1970s it moved from across the street into its present building, which had previously held P.S. 83, the first integrated school in New York City.

● Turn right on Schenectady Ave. and left on Bergen St. Another Weeksville church, Berean Baptist Church, is on your left after Utica Ave. The only extant Weeksville houses are on your right on the next block. They're known as the Hunterfly Road Houses, after the Indian trail turned country lane on which they were built. They were discovered amid overgrowth and behind Bergen St. rowhouses (since demolished) by a history teacher surveying the area from an airplane in 1968. Now restored, they're decorated to enlighten visitors about African-American family life and historical events in 1860, 1900, and 1930. Daily tours were initiated in June 2005, and within five years the Weeksville Heritage Center plans to add a large building for a museum, library, classrooms, and event space.

● Walk back to Utica and wait on the west side for the B46 bus to Kings Plaza. Take it to Eastern Pkwy., where you can transfer to the 3 or 4 train.

## POINTS OF INTEREST

**Jewish Children's Museum** 792 Eastern Pkwy., Brooklyn, NY 11213, 718-467-0600

**K&B Carib Kitchen** 268 Kingston Ave., Brooklyn, NY 11213, 718-363-1118

**Brower Park** Prospect Pl. between Brooklyn and Kingston Aves., Brooklyn, NY 11213

**Brooklyn Children's Museum** 145 Brooklyn Ave., Brooklyn, NY 11213, 718-735-4400

**Heru's Juice Bar** 111 Kingston Ave., Brooklyn, NY 11213, 718-756-9807

**Hunterfly Road Houses/Weeksville Heritage Center** 1698 Bergen St., Brooklyn, NY 11213, 718-756-5250

## ROUTE SUMMARY

1. Begin at Nostrand Ave. and President St. and walk east on President.
2. Turn left on Troy Ave., then left on Eastern Pkwy.
3. Turn right on New York Ave., then right on St. John's Pl.
4. Turn left on Brooklyn Ave.
5. Turn left on Park Pl.
6. Go right on New York Ave.
7. Turn right on Prospect Pl., walk through Brower Park, then go east on Park Pl. Turn left on Albany.
8. Go left on St. Mark's Ave.
9. Turn right on New York Ave.
10. Go right on Dean St., with a side trip down and back Kingston Ave.
11. Go right on Schenectady Ave. and left on Bergen St.
12. From the Hunterfly Road Houses, walk west on Bergen.
13. Get the southbound B46 bus on Utica Ave. and ride to Eastern Pkwy. for the subway.

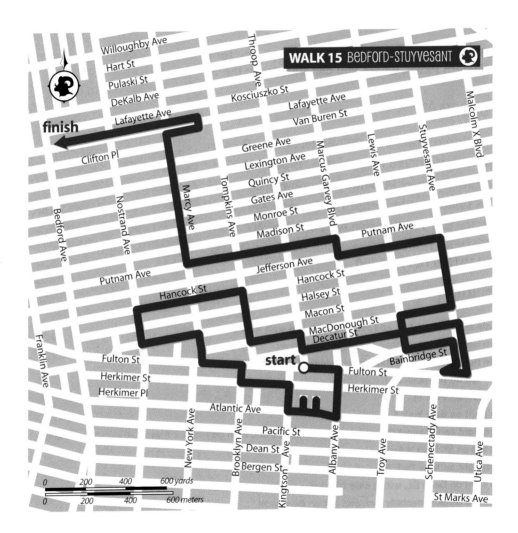

WALK 15 BeDFORD-STUYVeSANT

finish

Willoughby Ave
Hart St
Pulaski St
DeKalb Ave
Lafayette Ave
Clifton Pl

Throop Ave
Kosciuszko St
Lafayette Ave
Van Buren St

Greene Ave
Lexington Ave
Quincy St
Gates Ave
Monroe St
Madison St

Marcus Garvey Blvd
Lewis Ave
Stuyvesant Ave
Malcolm X Blvd

Marcy Ave
Tompkins Ave
Nostrand Ave
Bedford Ave

Putnam Ave
Putnam Ave

Jefferson Ave
Hancock St
Hancock St
Halsey St
Macon St
MacDonough St
Decatur St

Bainbridge St

start
Fulton St
Herkimer St

Franklin Ave
Fulton St
Herkimer St
Herkimer Pl

Atlantic Ave
Pacific St
Dean St
Bergen St

New York Ave
Brooklyn Ave
Kingston Ave
Albany Ave
Troy Ave
Schenectady Ave
Utica Ave

St Marks Ave

0    200    400    600 yards
0    200    400    600 meters

# 15 BeDForD-STUYVeSaNT: rooTS aND revivaL

**BOUNDARIES:** Atlantic Ave., Nostrand Ave., Lafayette Ave., Stuyvesant Ave.
**DISTANCE:** Approx. 5 miles
**SUBWAY:** C to Kingston–Throop Aves.

Bedford-Stuyvesant, the district that made history by electing the first black woman to the U.S. Congress (Shirley Chisholm), had become synonymous with "ghetto" by the 1970s. Comedian Chris Rock now jokes about his mid-'80s childhood in "Bed-Stuy: Do or Die." In New Yorker Billy Joel's 1980 song "You May Be Right," among the reckless behaviors mentioned: "I walked through Bedford-Stuy alone." This reputation has threatened to eclipse the neighborhood's architectural significance and profound African-American heritage. It possesses a bounty of Victorian homes built for the prosperous community of Stuyvesant Heights in the 1890s. That predominantly white area eventually merged with the larger, older, and more ethnically diverse town of Bedford, which had begun as a farming village in the 17th century. Blacks had a presence in Bedford almost from the beginning, but it became one of their prime destinations during the Great Migration. By some estimates, more blacks moved to Bed-Stuy than Harlem after the 1920s. Afrocentric cultural, religious, and social-service organizations have thrived here, and many of them have been involved in revitalization of the neighborhood over the last few decades.

- From the subway, walk east on Fulton St. and go right on Albany Ave.

- Turn right on Atlantic Ave., where the Long Island Rail Road runs on elevated tracks. Two picturesque cul-de-sacs have managed to evade the general drabness that's overtaken the area, just as they evaded the street grid that was implemented when Brooklyn became a city. Go in and out of Agate Ct. and Alice Ct. on your right, then continue west on Atlantic.

- Turn right on Kingston Ave. In 1833, a group of female reformers established the Brooklyn Orphans Asylum on the site of the playground to your left. It was a very progressive action in an era when the indigent were left to fend for themselves on the streets. The organization still exists as a foster-care agency.

● Turn left on Herkimer St., right on Brooklyn Ave., and left on Fulton St. Restoration Plaza, the retail and office complex on your left, was built in an old milk-bottling plant in the 1970s—a project of the Bedford Stuyvesant Restoration Corp., which spearheads housing, cultural, educational, and economic development initiatives for the neighborhood. It was cofounded in 1967 by Robert F. Kennedy (then a U.S. senator representing New York) and is the oldest community-development corporation in the country. Within Restoration Plaza, the Billie Holiday Theatre's resident company produces new works by black playwrights.

● Turn right on Marcy Ave. and left on Macon St. As you near Nostrand Ave., you are walking beside the 1912 addition to Girls' High School. At Nostrand, you can see all of this fabulous building, the oldest public secondary-school building in New York City. It opened in 1886 and is the alma mater of Shirley Chisholm and Lena Horne. Across from it is the Alhambra, the older (and more sensational) of two sumptuous Nostrand Ave. dwellings designed by Montrose Morris. The first major commission for Morris, a Bedford resident who became one of Brooklyn's most influential residential architects, the Alhambra contained 30 nine-room apartments when it opened in 1889. Be sure to see the building from all three sides, on Macon, Nostrand, and Halsey.

● Across Halsey St. on Nostrand is the Renaissance, Morris's 1892 masterstroke. Here he opted for a French chateau paradigm, banded the brick and terra cotta, and rounded the corner towers (as opposed to the Alhambra's polygons).

● Turn right on Hancock St. Proceed from the tall brownstones between Nostrand and Marcy to a block filled with Morris's pre-Alhambra output, starting with the Queen Anne enchantress at 232 Hancock St. on your right at the corner with Marcy. The house at #236 was both his residence and his marketing medium—he created it to show prospective clients what he was capable of. He also designed #244–#252 and #255–#259. Many consider the freestanding brownstone at #247 to be the belle of the block.

● Turn right on Tompkins Ave. Two brick houses of worship from the 1880s face each other on your right at MacDonough St. The more prominent in both history and size is First AME Zion Church, with a campanile like that of St. Mark's in Venice. The Congregationalists who built the church had more worshippers than any other congregation of their denomination in the United States. Across the street, Stuyvesant Heights Christian Church boasts large stained-glass windows.

- Turn left on MacDonough. From 1888 to 1988, the detached house to the left of #97 was a local branch of the United Order of Tents, a lodge for African-American women founded in Virginia by two slaves and two abolitionists. Aside from a small row of homes with Spanish-tile roofs, classic brownstones dominate the block.

- At Throop Ave., the limestone-trimmed Our Lady of Victory Catholic Church (1891–95) spans the east side of the street north of MacDonough. But turn right to walk south on Throop. If you desire refreshment, go one more block on MacDonough to Marcus Garvey Blvd. and Food 4 Thought, a juice bar/café with a social conscience and artistic spirit. Then backtrack to Throop and walk south.

- Turn left on Decatur St. Among this street's elegant residences are the Clermont apartments at #79–#81, built in 1900 and ornamented with fleurs-de-lis. There's a pocket park on your right at Albany Ave. Decatur's late-19th-century churches include Bethany Baptist, on your left at Marcus Garvey Blvd., and Mount Lebanon Baptist, on your right across Lewis Ave.

- Go right on Stuyvesant Ave. and then right at Chauncey St. Across from a superb row of townhouses, enter Fulton Park—which was named after Fulton St., its southern boundary, rather than steamboat inventor Robert Fulton (though the street was of course named after him). The statue of Fulton was erected on the waterfront in 1872, when ferries were still the only way to travel between Brooklyn and Manhattan. It disappeared after the ferry house

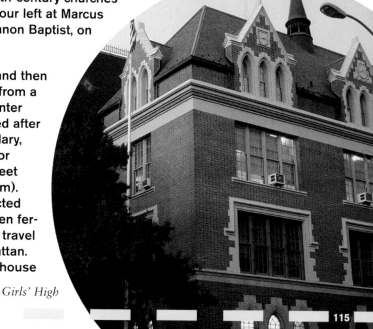

*Girls' High*

115

was torn down in 1926, and when it was finally recovered it only made sense to put it in a park named Fulton. Badly deteriorated, the statue had to be recast in bronze in 1955. A garden lies ahead of Mr. Fulton at the tip of the triangular park. Exit near the pavilion and go left on Stuyvesant.

● Turn left on Bainbridge St., an attractive block with an entertaining assortment of designs on your right and straitlaced homes on your left.

● Turn right on Lewis. You may wish to browse in Brownstone Books at Decatur. Then go right on MacDonough. The Gothic church on your right with gargoyles perched from the tallest pinnacle was constructed in 1899. Since 1944 it has been home to St. Philip's Episcopal, a congregation founded in Weeksville, a community within Bedford (now Crown Heights) established by blacks after slavery was abolished. St. Philip's sponsored the first black Boy Scout troop in the country. Mansions on the block include the Akwaaba B&B at #347, an 1860 villa fully restored in 1995 by Monique Greenwood, then editor in chief of *Essence* magazine, and her husband, Glenn Pogue. There's a community garden at the corner on your left.

● Turn left on Stuyvesant. Bridge Street African Wesleyan Methodist Episcopal Church, on your right at Jefferson Ave., is the oldest black congregation in Brooklyn, founded in 1818 and named for the street in Downtown where its previous church was located. The church spends about half its income on housing renovation and construction and runs a school, credit union, apartment buildings, and senior citizens center.

● Go left on Jefferson. After crossing Lewis, you time-travel from the Victorian era to the Middle Ages. All that's missing is a moat around the castle (maybe that would keep it graffiti-free). The castle, which is on your right, was the 13th Regiment Armory. Walk alongside it, then turn right on Marcus Garvey Blvd. to see it from the front. As with several other colossal National Guard armories built in the late 1800s, construction of this one incited allegations of patronage and pork barreling. Its $700,000 final cost was more than twice what had been allotted, and the watchtower had to be reduced in height.

● From Marcus Garvey Blvd., turn left on Putnam Ave. Then turn right on Marcy Ave., with Boys' High School in front of you. This male counterpart to Girls' High School down on Nostrand was built in 1891 and counted Isaac Asimov, Norman Mailer, and Aaron Copland among its graduates. Across Marcy at Madison St., Concord Baptist is one of the country's largest black churches, with 12,000 members, an excellent choir, 160 years of history, and an active role in local political and social issues. Be sure to see its high entryway and rose window on Madison. Continuing on Marcy, you come to St. George's Episcopal (1887) at Gates Ave., then Herbert Von King Park at Greene Ave. Initially named Tompkins, it's Bed-Stuy's largest and one of Brooklyn's earliest parks and was designed by Frederick Law Olmsted and Calvert Vaux (who did Prospect Park and Central Park). Impressionist painter William Merritt Chase, an Indiana native, lived nearby on Marcy and painted Tompkins in *A City Park.*

● Stay on Marcy to see the Hattie Carthan Garden at Clifton Pl., then turn right on Lafayette Ave. to visit local environmentalist Carthan's pet project across from the park: the Magnolia Grandiflora. A seedling from North Carolina was planted in 1885, and the fragrant state flower of Louisiana and Mississippi has been growing in Brooklyn ever since. The city granted landmark status to the tree and the houses next to it, since they protect it from north winds. The Magnolia Tree Earth Center is an environmental and cultural organization that sprung up around the tree, and Carthan is memorialized in a mural next to it.

● Turn around and walk west on Lafayette to the Bedford Ave. station of the G train.

## POINTS OF INTEREST

**Food 4 Thought** 445 Marcus Garvey Blvd., Brooklyn, NY 11216, 718-443-4160

**Fulton Park** Chauncey St. between Lewis and Stuyvesant Aves., Brooklyn, NY 11233

**Brownstone Books** 409 Lewis Ave., Brooklyn, NY 11233, 718-953-7328

**Akwaaba Mansion** 347 MacDonough St., Brooklyn, NY 11233, 718-455-5958

**Herbert Von King Park** Greene Ave. between Marcy and Tompkins Aves., Brooklyn, NY 11216

**Magnolia Tree Earth Center** 677 Lafayette Ave., Brooklyn, NY 11216, 718-387-2116

# route summary

1. From Fulton St. and Throop Ave., walk east on Fulton and turn right on Albany Ave.

2. Turn right on Atlantic Ave. to visit Agate and Alice Cts.

3. Turn right on Kingston Ave.

4. Turn left on Herkimer St., right on Brooklyn Ave., and left on Fulton.

5. Turn right on Marcy Ave., then left on Macon St.

6. Turn right on Nostrand Ave.

7. Go right on Hancock St.

8. Go right on Tompkins Ave.

9. Turn left on MacDonough St.

10. Turn right on Throop.

11. Go left on Decatur St.

12. Turn right on Stuyvesant Ave., then right at Chauncey St. and into Fulton Park.

13. Walk north from the park on Stuyvesant to Bainbridge St. and turn left.

14. Turn right on Lewis Ave., then right on MacDonough.

15. Turn left on Stuyvesant.

16. Turn left on Jefferson Ave., then right on Marcus Garvey Blvd.

17. Turn left on Putnam Ave., then right on Marcy.

18. Go right on Lafayette Ave. to visit the magnolia tree.

19. Turn around and walk west on Lafayette to the subway.

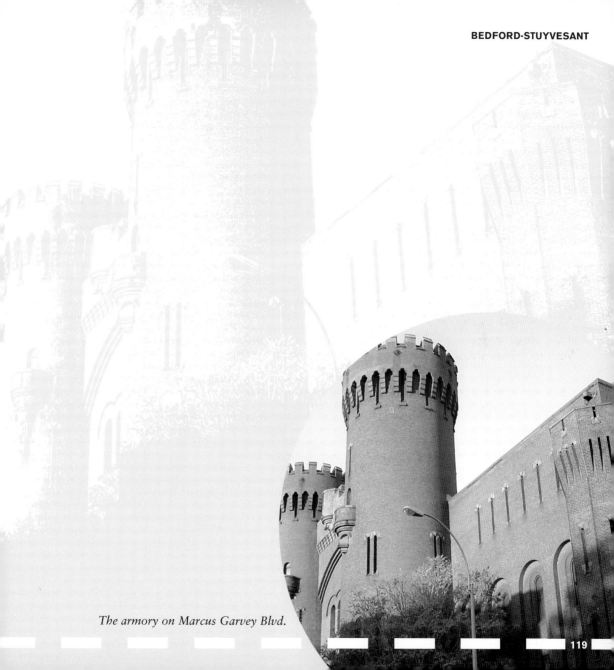

*The armory on Marcus Garvey Blvd.*

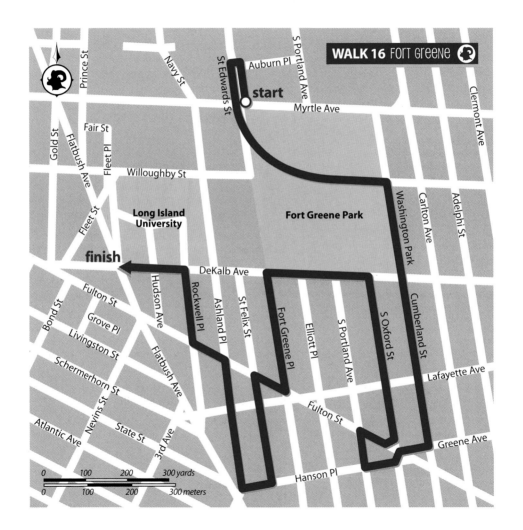

**WALK 16** Fort Greene

Prince St

Navy St

St Edwards St

Auburn Pl

S Portland Ave

**start**

Myrtle Ave

Clermont Ave

Fair St

Gold St

Flatbush Ave

Fleet Pl

Willoughby St

Fleet St

Washington Park

Carlton Ave

Adelphi St

**Long Island University**

**Fort Greene Park**

**finish**

DeKalb Ave

Hudson Ave

Rockwell Pl

Ashland Pl

St Felix St

Fort Greene Pl

Elliott Pl

S Portland Ave

S Oxford St

Cumberland St

Fulton St

Bond St

Grove Pl

Livingston St

Schermerhorn St

Flatbush Ave

Lafayette Ave

Atlantic Ave

Nevins St

State St

3rd Ave

Fulton St

Greene Ave

Hanson Pl

| 0 | 100 | 200 | 300 yards |
| 0 | 100 | 200 | 300 meters |

# 16 Fort Greene: Gaze Up, Look Back, Search Within

**BOUNDARIES: Auburn Pl., Cumberland St., Hanson Pl., Rockwell Pl.**
**DISTANCE: Approx. 2¼ miles**
**SUBWAY: A, C, or F to Jay St.–Borough Hall, transfer to B54 bus to Ridgewood**

Fort Greene has earned many bragging rights. It's home to Brooklyn's only skyscraper, the 512-foot-tall Williamsburgh Savings Bank tower. It has the oldest performing-arts institution in the country, the still-vibrant Brooklyn Academy of Music. It has one of the city's most profound memorials, located within a park designed by Frederick Law Olmsted and Calvert Vaux. And a great American novel, Richard Wright's *Native Son,* was written here. In fact, Fort Greene is a source of pride for African-Americans (two-thirds of the neighborhood's population) in many respects—from its cultural energy to its eluding the ghettoization that befell other black Brooklyn neighborhoods like East New York and Bushwick. Since its post-agricultural development, this has been a middle-class neighborhood, with a wealth of scenic, cultural, and historic treasures.

● Get off the bus on Myrtle Ave. at St. Edwards St. Cross Myrtle, and you're beside the Walt Whitman housing project, which, along with the adjacent Ingersoll Houses, was built by the city for World War II–era employees of the Brooklyn Navy Yard, located just a few blocks north. They may not look it, but Whitman and Ingersoll were designed by several of NYC's premier architects of the time. Walk on St. Edwards to see three noteworthy buildings within the complex. First, on your left, is St. Michael and St. Edward, a 100-year-old church that bears some resemblance to a chateau. Cross Auburn Pl. Of the 58 branches of the Brooklyn Public Library, this one on your right carries the name of the greatest literary figure associated with the borough, Walt Whitman. The brick building dates to 1907 and was paid for by Andrew Carnegie. P.S. 67, next to the library, is where formal education began for the black population of Brooklyn. It opened in 1847 as Colored School No. 1, serving a student body composed of the children of freed slaves (many of whom were employed at the Navy Yard).

- Turn back on St. Edwards in the direction you came, recross Myrtle, and enter Fort Greene Park—30 acres of greenery and play areas on the Revolutionary War site of Fort Putnam. The park was established in 1847 after campaigning by *Brooklyn Eagle* editor Walt Whitman, who was concerned about ample breathing room for crowded city dwellers. A formal design by landscape architects Frederick Law Olmsted and Calvert Vaux was implemented in 1867 following the pair's success with Central Park. Take the path to the left, walking between a playground and basketball courts, then begin ascending the steps of the Prison Ship Martyrs Memorial. During the American Revolution, approximately 11,500 prisoners of war perished aboard British ships docked in Wallabout Bay (which was landfilled to build the Navy Yard)—a death toll almost three times as great as the combat casualties.

- Before the top set of steps, leave the staircase via the path on your right. On the lawn to your left, look for the four trees with whiter trunks—they're 150-year-old London planes, planted here in the Olmsted/Vaux design. Proceed to the paved plaza next to the trees. Richard Wright lived a block away (at 175 Carlton Ave.) when he was writing *Native Son,* but did most of the writing on this hill mornings from 6:00 to 10:00 A.M. The bench in the plaza is dedicated to Wright. Bend down to see quotations from *Native Son* imprinted on its legs.

- Take the path across the staircase to the other side of the Prison Ship Martyrs Memorial and go inside the visitors center, housed in a 1908 mini-temple that may have been the last thing designed by architect Stanford White (the memorial's architect) before he was murdered by his mistress's husband in one of the city's all-time most-buzzed-about scandals.

- Leave the park via the path to your left out of the visitors center. You'll be on Washington Park, a splendid street of 1880s brownstones (houses at #173 to #186 date to the 1860s). Go to your right. Across DeKalb Ave., the street becomes Cumberland St. On your right, look for #260, the 1929–65 home of Pulitzer Prize–winning poet Marianne Moore, a native Missourian who was a civic activist in her adopted hometown and one of the Dodger faithful.

- Take Cumberland to the right into Cuyler Gore, a triangular park (that's what "gore" means) named for abolitionist minister Theodore Ledyard Cuyler, who humbly declined to have a statue erected of himself—he considered the park honor enough.

- Turn right on the path midway into the park and exit at the tip of the triangle where Fulton St. and Greene Ave. meet. Cross Fulton and turn right on Hanson Pl. At the next corner, on your left will be Hanson Place Seventh Day Adventist Church, a city landmark whose grandeur comes not only from its striking exterior but from what took place out of sight of passersby: before the church was built in 1860, the property was part of the Underground Railroad.

- Across S. Portland Ave., visit MoCADA, the Museum of Contemporary African Diasporan Arts, which moved to these new quarters from Bedford-Stuyvesant in 2006.

- Cross Hanson Pl. and proceed on S. Portland the short block to Fulton St., and turn right. That burst of color across the street is Habana Outpost, the Brooklyn offshoot of Manhattan's Café Habana, which itself was modeled after Mexico City's Café Habana. A Mexican-Cuban menu shares top billing with environmental sustainability at this "eco-eatery," which uses solar and wind power, purchases organic ingredients from regional growers, and made its patio tables out of recycled material. It supports neighborhood artists by hosting performances and craft markets on the premises.

- Turn left on S. Oxford St. The tall brown tower belongs to Lafayette Avenue Presbyterian Church, where Reverend Cuyler—remember the gore?—was pastor for 30 years commencing with its 1862 opening. This church was also a stop on the

*Williamsburgh Savings Bank's clocktower*

## THE PARAMOUNT LIVES ON

Inside the building at the northeast corner of Flatbush and DeKalb Aves., across the street from the subway station where you end the Fort Greene walk, are probably the most stunning school gym and student union you're likely to see. They're part of Long Island University, which was lucky enough to incorporate the former Paramount theater into its Brooklyn campus and smart enough to preserve the spectacular interior. The Paramount thrived from 1928 to 1962, before cookie-cutter multiplexes displaced opulent movie palaces. Its fountains and colored lights are long gone, but not the carved wood ceiling and Wurlitzer organ (now in the gym) or the two-story lobby with grand staircase, columns, and marble walls (now overlooking a cafeteria). The Paramount could seat over 4,000 patrons, who flocked to the theater not only for movies but also for live shows. Earlier generations saw such talents as George Gershwin and Ethel Merman on the Paramount stage, and in the 1950s deejay Alan Freed presented the first-ever rock-and-roll concerts there. How to get inside without a university ID? Call 718-488-1000 to try to arrange a visit, or go during a home game of the Brooklyn Kings minor-league basketball team, or just sweet-talk the security guard into letting you take a quick peek.

Underground Railroad. Cuyler was known nationwide (even by Abraham Lincoln) for his antislavery activism but nonetheless was censured by Presbyterian authorities for allowing a woman to preach at the church. When Sarah Smiley, a Quaker, addressed the LAPC congregation at Cuyler's invitation in 1872, she became the first woman ever to preach from a Presbyterian pulpit.

● Continue on S. Oxford. Across Lafayette Ave., two eye-catching apartment houses face each other as you enter the brownstone block. On the right is the Roanoke, built in 1893 in Romanesque Revival style; on the left, the Griffin, an Art Deco former hotel from the early 1930s.

● Turn left on DeKalb and pop in at the Greene Garden on your left between S. Portland and S. Elliott Pl. (open to the public on Tuesdays, Thursdays, weekends, and unscheduled "other times"). The garden resembles a backyard nirvana—right down to its little Buddha statue.

- Before turning left on Fort Greene Pl., look ahead on DeKalb: that red banner with 40A in a circle hangs from a former firehouse that's home to 40 Acres and a Mule Filmworks, director Spike Lee's production company. Lee lived in Fort Greene for a while and shot his breakout film, *She's Gotta Have It,* in the park.

- At the Fulton/Lafayette nexus with Fort Greene Pl. is another little triangular park. Turn right on Fulton St., then left around the park to find its entrance at Lafayette and St. Felix St.

- Across St. Felix on Lafayette is the Brooklyn Academy of Music, and could anything be more welcoming than the musician cherubs around the doorways? BAM (pronounced as one syllable) boasts a 2,000-seat opera house whose ceiling is gilded like a Faberge egg; a ballroom with 24-foot-high windows, now used as a cafe; and a four-screen cinema. Tantamount to its physical splendor is BAM's artistic legacy—from Enrico Caruso's penultimate performance to the annual New Wave Festival, an acclaimed showcase for new and avant-garde works.

- Walk down St. Felix. On your right, the Brooklyn Music School and Playhouse is another linchpin of Fort Greene's cultural district, offering performing arts classes since 1912; it recently took in a resident theater company, the Sackett Group.

- Turn right on Hanson Pl., and find another of Fort Greene's claims to fame as you turn right onto Ashland Pl.: the 1929 Williamsburgh Savings Bank tower, sometimes referred to simply as the clocktower, since the bank no longer exists. The critters depicted in the exterior embossments are symbols of thrift, ironic given the extravagant price tags of the apartments inside. Do go inside the former bank lobby at street level if you can to fully appreciate this landmark's magnificence.

- From Ashland, turn left on Fulton to see BAM's addition, the Harvey Theater (named after executive director Harvey Lichtenstein, who spearheaded the institution's renaissance during his 1967–99 tenure). It still displays the 1903 theater's earlier name, Majestic, because when BAM took over the performance space it restored but did not overlay any part of the structure inside or out. At the corner with Rockwell Pl., another old theater, the Strand, has been adapted for use by another Fort Greene–based arts organization, Brooklyn Information & Culture (BRIC), which has a cable-access TV studio and black-box theater inside. While the old Strand's Latin inscriptions are vintage, the fading painted signage on the Rockwell side of the building—parking for 25¢—is even more of a classic.

● Turn right on Rockwell to visit yet another creative enterprise: Urban Glass, where you can watch craftspeople at work through a viewing window in the shop, which sells items made by artists affiliated with the studio. There's also a gallery for exhibits of glass art.

● At DeKalb, the soul-food restaurant Ruthies to your right is a neighborhood institution. The B/Q/R trains are a couple of blocks in the other direction on DeKalb.

## POINTS OF INTEREST

**Brooklyn Public Library–Walt Whitman** 93 St. Edwards St., Brooklyn, NY 11205, 718-935-0244

**Fort Greene Park** Myrtle Ave. between St. Edwards St. and Washington Park, Brooklyn, NY 11217

**MoCADA** 80 Hanson Pl. (on S. Portland Ave.), Brooklyn, NY 11217, 718-230-0492

**Habana Outpost** 757 Fulton St., Brooklyn, NY 11217, 718-858-9500

**Greene Garden** DeKalb Ave. between S. Portland Ave. and S. Elliott Pl., Brooklyn, NY 11217

**Brooklyn Academy of Music** 30 Lafayette Ave., Brooklyn, NY 11217, 718-636-4100

**Sackett Group** 126 St. Felix St., Brooklyn, NY 11217, 718-638-7104

**Williamsburgh Savings Bank** 1 Hanson Pl., Brooklyn, NY 11217

**Brooklyn Information & Culture (BRIC)** 647 Fulton St., Brooklyn, NY 11217, 718-855-7882

**Urban Glass** 57 Rockwell Pl., Brooklyn, NY 11217, 718-625-3685

**Ruthies** 96 DeKalb Ave., Brooklyn, NY 11201, 718-246-5189

# route summary

1. Begin on Myrtle Ave. at St. Edwards St.
2. Turn left on St. Edwards, proceed past Auburn Pl., then turn around and go back to Myrtle.
3. Enter Fort Greene Park and walk through it up the hill.
4. Exit the park on Washington Park and go to the right. Washington Park becomes Cumberland St.
5. Enter Cuyler Gore from Cumberland, turn right, and leave the park at Greene Ave. and Fulton St.
6. Turn right on Hanson Pl.
7. Turn right on S. Portland Ave., then right on Fulton.
8. Turn left on S. Oxford St.
9. Turn left on DeKalb Ave.
10. Turn left on Fort Greene Pl.
11. Turn right on Fulton.
12. Turn left on St. Felix St.
13. Turn right on Hanson Pl. and right on Ashland Pl.
14. Turn left on Fulton, then right on Rockwell Pl.
15. Turn left on DeKalb to get to the subway (or go right for Ruthies first).

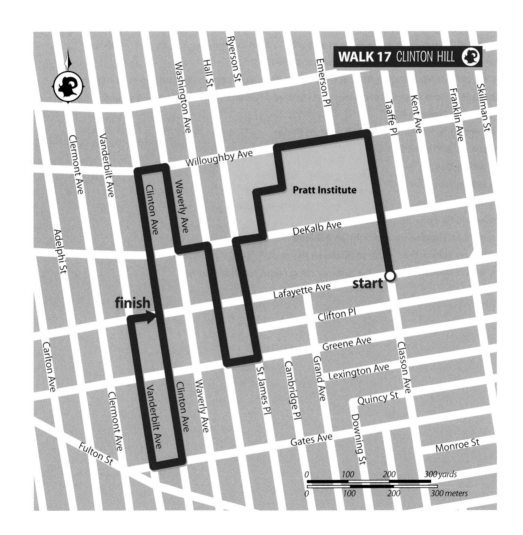

WALK 17 CLINTON HILL

Pratt Institute

Willoughby Ave
DeKalb Ave
Lafayette Ave
Clifton Pl
Greene Ave
Lexington Ave
Quincy St
Gates Ave
Monroe St
Fulton St

Ryerson St
Emerson Pl
Taaffe Pl
Kent Ave
Franklin Ave
Skillman St
Hall St
Washington Ave
Clermont Ave
Vanderbilt Ave
Adelphi St
Clinton Ave
Waverly Ave
Carlton Ave
Clermont Ave
St James Pl
Cambridge Pl
Grand Ave
Classon Ave
Downing St

start

finish

0    100    200    300 yards
0    100    200    300 meters

# 17 CLINTON HILL: POSH ENCLAVE TURNED COLLEGE TOWN

**BOUNDARIES: Classon Ave., Willoughby Ave., Vanderbilt Ave., Gates Ave.**
**DISTANCE: Approx. 1¾ miles**
**SUBWAY: G to Classon Ave.**

In the late 19th century, Clinton Hill was the most prestigious address in Brooklyn after Brooklyn Heights. Charles Pratt, Brooklyn's wealthiest resident and the owner of Greenpoint-based Astral Oil, put the neighborhood on the map when he moved into his brand-new mansion in 1875. A number of Pratt's fellow tycoons, some of whose names we know today from the companies they founded, followed Pratt to "the Hill"—among them, Messrs. Pfizer, Bristol, and Liebmann (owner of the Rheingold brewery). Pratt built more houses on his block for his sons to live in after they married, and he helped fund other construction in the area. His biggest project was Pratt Institute, a design and engineering college whose pretty campus doubles as a top-notch sculpture garden.

- The first things you'll see when you exit the subway at Classon and Lafayette Aves. are high-rise apartment buildings, a playground, and a couple of convenience stores. Looks like any old urban neighborhood, huh? You're in for a surprise! "Old" maybe, but not "any old." With the playground on your left, walk north on Classon. On your left at the corner with DeKalb Ave. is the New York Police Department's 88th Precinct, housed in a vine-covered 1890 brick building with a high conical tower.

- Turn left on Willoughby Ave. The green-steepled church on your right is St. Mary's Episcopal, a Gothic Revival construction from 1859. After you cross Emerson Pl., there are slightly scruffy rowhouses with alternating tops of red brick in a step shape (so-called Dutch style) and triangular mock Tudor facing. These are among the nearly 30 rowhouses the Pratt family built on Willoughby, Emerson, and Steuben—some of the streets bordering the Pratt Institute campus.

- Enter Pratt through the main gate opposite Grand Ave. Follow along as described, or wander on your own: each building and work of art has a marker and campus maps are prominently posted, so self-navigating is easy.

- From the Grand Ave. path, look across the grass on your left at the backside of a 30-foot reclining human figure made of cement on steel. Other sculptures on the lawn include a playful interpretation of a rock garden. On the other side of the path stands one of the first buildings constructed for the school. Now called the East Building and formerly known as the Machine Shop—note the smokestack—it contains the oldest steam-powered generators still in use in the Northeast. Go into the building through the door with an intertwined P and I above it for a look at this extraordinary power plant. You'll also see assorted obsolete industrial pieces, and you'll probably encounter at least one of the Pratt Cats. Ribbons they've earned at cat shows over the years are on display, as is information about their role in the campus community.

- Exit the building at the other end of the corridor. You'll be in a courtyard, and at its center is a trickling fountain carved with a forest scene and mythological figures. Take the steps to your left, which lead through the semicircular bleachers of a small amphitheater.

- Go to the right on the paths to Ryerson Walk. On your right are three adjoining Romanesque edifices. The Main Hall in the middle was built, like the Machine Shop, when the school opened in 1887. A few years later came South Hall, whose architect then created the porch for the Main Hall. Memorial Hall was added to the campus in the 1920s (a plaque incorrectly says that both South and Memorial are from the '20s).

- Across Ryerson Walk and up a few steps you'll find a rose garden—most noticeable, obviously, when it's in bloom—and several outsize sculptures, as well as two steel tiger skeletons engaged in combat.

- Pratt's library, an 1896 building just south of the roses and tigers, was originally a public library—the first free one in Brooklyn, in fact. Continuing south on Ryerson Walk, look to your right for two huge white fiberglass heads (named Victoria and Eucantha) and a series of feet—Brancusi's feet, in honor of the abstract innovator who walked from his native Romania to Paris to become an artist.

- Next to the gate at the end of Ryerson Walk is Robert Indiana's iconic pop-art *LOVE*, which was used on a postage stamp. Leave the campus through this gate on DeKalb

Ave. and go to your right. At St. James Pl. you can grab a bite at Mike's Coffee Shop, a classic old luncheonette serving Pratt students.

● Turn left on St. James. At Lafayette Ave., check out Emmanuel Baptist Church (inside if possible)—built in 1887 and paid for by Charles Pratt, a devout Baptist. Across Lafayette on the other side of St. James are two Romanesque Revival buildings, the north one erected in 1867 and the south one about 20 years later (on Charles Pratt's dime). The buildings, now part of Pratt Institute, were the original campus of the Adelphi prep school and college.

● Turn right on Greene Ave. and right on Washington Ave. The gorgeous building on your right at #379 had, believe it or not, deteriorated into a seedy hotel before being restored in the 1980s as fashionable apartment living. On Washington at Lafayette, Underwood Park is named for the typewriter mogul whose mansion once stood here. Next to the park, the rehabbed apartment building at 320 Washington Ave. is still inscribed GRAHAM HOME FOR OLD LADIES—a now laughably indelicate name that reveals only part of the place's history. The home opened in 1851 and operated for over a century. After it closed, the building deteriorated into a fleabag hotel occupied by other kinds of ladies (of the evening).

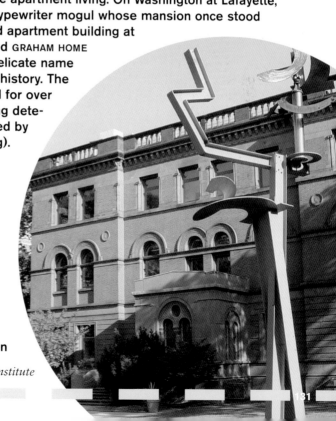

● Turn left on DeKalb and right on Waverly Ave., narrower and subtler than neighboring Washington and Clinton Aves. since it held the carriage houses and stables for those avenues' mansions.

● Turn left on Willoughby and left on Clinton, where you will enjoy four blocks of stunning residential architecture in various styles. The most famous homes, sitting between

*The library and a sculpture at Pratt Institute*

## OPEN STUDIO WEEKENDS

Clinton Hill, like other communities in western Brooklyn, is populated with artists. And many Clinton Hill artists participate in the springtime Studio Stroll sponsored by the organization South of the Navy Yard Artists. SONYA is just one Brooklyn artist group that runs an annual open studio weekend. Artists open up their studios—which often are also their homes—to visitors, who get to chat with the artists and observe the creative process close-up. No entrance fees are charged. Open studio weekends take place on spring and autumn weekends, and sponsoring organizations provide maps of participating locations.

The SONYA Studio Stroll, which is held the third weekend of May, entails Fort Greene and Bedford-Stuyvesant in addition to Clinton Hill. Also held in mid- to late May is the Park Slope and Environs Artists Open Studio Tour, which features free van transportation between sites (those "environs" extend to Boerum Hill, Windsor Terrace, and Sunset Park).

There are two open studio events in early June: the Atlantic Avenue ArtWalk in Boerum Hill and Cobble Hill, and the Brooklyn Waterfront Artists Coalition's Open Studio Weekend in Red Hook and Carroll Gardens. Open studios are part of the Art Under the Bridge Festival in Dumbo every October. Around the same time, the Annual Gowanus Artists Studio Tour takes place in Gowanus and the western fringes of Park Slope.

Willoughby and DeKalb, belonged to the Pratt family. Charles lived at #232, which is now Founders Hall of St. Joseph's College, and built the mansions across the street for his sons as wedding presents: the Georgian-style #245 was the last to go up, in 1901; stately #241 beside it had been the first in 1890 and today is the Roman Catholic bishop of Brooklyn's residence. The most alluring of the Pratt homes, #229, suggests a villa with its arbored second-floor terrace lined with busts. But my favorite house on this block is quirky #278, with its two types of windows and two different balconies. The house at #284 dates all the way back to the 1850s.

● Turn right on Gates Ave. The Royal Castle on your left was built with much Beaux Arts flourish around 1911 and still rates as one of the city's finest apartment houses.

- Turn right on Vanderbilt Ave. A meticulous row of 1880s Italianate brownstones stretches out on your left. When you reach Lafayette Ave., look across to your left at two ornate century-old structures. The church with over 20 statues and horizontal gargoyles is Queen of All Saints; next to it is the Brooklyn Masonic Temple, built in a Classical style and admired for its brown-and-white terra cotta detail.

- Turn right on Lafayette. At the corner on your right is a yellow clapboard house with white trim. Its smaller eastern wing may look like an annex, but that section dates to 1812, making the house one of the oldest in Brooklyn (the rest of it is from the 1850s). Referred to by the names of both recent and previous occupants, the house is variously known as the Joseph Steele or Steele-Brick-Skinner House.

- There's a G subway station at Lafayette and Clinton.

## POINTS OF INTEREST

**Pratt Institute** 200 Willoughby Ave., Brooklyn, NY 11205, 718-636-3600
**Mike's Coffee Shop** 328 DeKalb Ave., Brooklyn, NY 11205, 718-857-1462
**Underwood Park** Washington and Lafayette Aves., Brooklyn, NY 11205

## route summary

1. Begin at Classon and Lafayette Aves. and walk north on Classon.
2. Turn left on Willoughby Ave.
3. Enter Pratt Institute and tour the campus. Exit on DeKalb Ave. and go right.
4. Turn left on St. James Pl.
5. Turn right on Greene Ave. and right on Washington Ave.
6. Turn left on DeKalb and right on Waverly Ave.
7. Turn left on Willoughby Ave. and left on Clinton Ave.
8. Turn right on Gates Ave.
9. Turn right on Vanderbilt Ave.
10. Turn right on Lafayette back to Clinton and the subway.

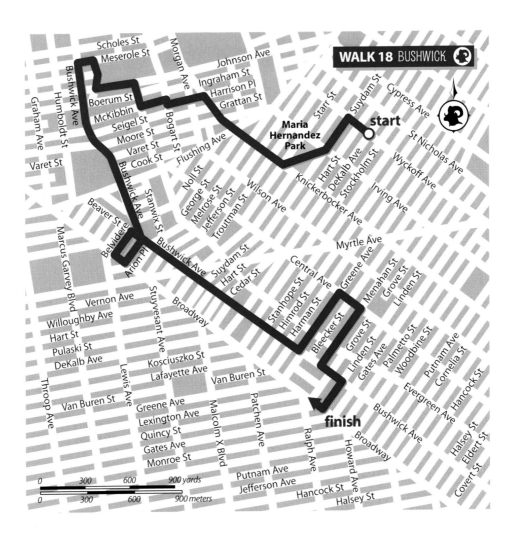

**WALK 18** BUSHWICK

start

finish

Maria Hernandez Park

Scholes St
Meserole St
Morgan Ave
Johnson Ave
Ingraham St
Harrison Pl
Grattan St
Boerum St
McKibbin
Seigel St
Moore St
Varet St
Cook St
Bushwick Ave
Humboldt St
Graham Ave
Varet St
Bogart St
Flushing Ave
Noll St
George St
Melrose St
Jefferson St
Troutman St
Wilson Ave
Starr St
Suydam St
Cypress Ave
St Nicholas Ave
Wyckoff Ave
Hart St
DeKalb Ave
Stockholm St
Knickerbocker Ave
Irving Ave
Beaver St
Belvidere
Stanwix St
Bushwick Ave
Arion Pl
Marcus Garvey Blvd
Vernon Ave
Willoughby Ave
Hart St
Pulaski St
DeKalb Ave
Stuyvesant Ave
Broadway
Suydam St
Hart St
Cedar St
Myrtle Ave
Greene Ave
Menahan St
Grove St
Linden St
Central Ave
Stanhope St
Himrod St
Harman St
Bleecker St
Grove St
Linden St
Gates St
Palmetto St
Woodbine St
Putnam Ave
Cornelia St
Evergreen Ave
Hancock St
Throop Ave
Lewis Ave
Van Buren St
Greene Ave
Lexington Ave
Quincy St
Gates Ave
Monroe St
Kosciuszko St
Lafayette Ave
Van Buren St
Malcolm X Blvd
Patchen Ave
Putnam Ave
Jefferson Ave
Ralph Ave
Howard Ave
Bushwick Ave
Broadway
Hancock St
Halsey St
Halsey St
Eldert St
Covert St

0   300   600   900 yards
0   300   600   900 meters

# 18 BUSHWICK: ALONG THE BEER BARONS' BOULEVARD

**BOUNDARIES:** Wyckoff Ave., Meserole St., Broadway, Linden St.
**DISTANCE:** Approx. 4 miles
**SUBWAY:** L to DeKalb Ave.

In tracing the history of Bushwick, one of the five original Kings County towns founded by the Dutch (as Boswijck in 1661), two words are bound to come up: beer and blackout. Bushwick's brewing industry, which before Prohibition accounted for 1 in 10 beers drunk in the country, may have begun with Hessian soldiers who stuck around after aiding the king's army in the Battle of Brooklyn, but it burgeoned in the mid-1800s, when thousands of German immigrants moved in. After World War II, Bushwick started losing both its economic linchpin and middle-class stability. Beer companies consolidated production at plants outside New York, and families fled to the suburbs. The biggest blow occurred in July 1977, when looters and arsonists laid siege to ghettos like Bushwick during a 26-hour citywide blackout. By the time the lights came on, some 35 blocks in Bushwick had been nearly destroyed and $300 million in damage done. Within a year, 40 percent of businesses shuttered; the population fell by more than 20 percent by the end of the decade. Bushwick's woes persisted through the '80s with the crack epidemic. In the mid-'90s, community social-service initiatives and low-income housing improvements set Bushwick on an upswing. Though still one of the city's poorest districts, Bushwick is now being pegged as the next place for hipsters to colonize when they're priced out of neighboring Williamsburg. Some have started calling it East Williamsburg.

● When you exit the subway at DeKalb Ave., look for the Empire State Building and walk in its direction on Wyckoff Ave. You're two blocks from the border with Queens.

● Turn left on Suydam St. At Irving Ave., enter Maria Hernandez Park, the community's recreational hub. Read the history of the park (it involves P.T. Barnum) in the sign on the comfort station; one thing it doesn't tell you is that two drug dealers were convicted of Maria Hernandez's murder. Take the path to your right, pausing if you're musically inclined to tinker with one of the human-size instruments—xylophone and conga drums—among the swings in the playground. Leave the park at the corner of Starr St. and Knickerbocker Ave. and go right on Knickerbocker. You can get some authentic Latino food here—Alex Aguinaga, for example, is a homey Ecuadoran restaurant, on your left past Troutman. Knickerbocker's many Latino businesses include a few record stores usually playing music for passersby.

- Past Flushing Ave., you enter East Williamsburg Industrial Park, where artists and small manufacturers work in renovated warehouse lofts. From this part of Knickerbocker, you also have a nice view of the Midtown skyline, framed by the Chrysler Building and slanty-roofed Citicorp Center.

- Turn left on Harrison Pl., right on Bogart St., and left on McKibbin St. Opposite a concrete manufacturer that's open to the public (?!), go left into Justice Gilbert Ramirez Park, which features funky-shaped swings, replicas of subway lampposts and signage, and a metal mural of street scenes. Exit at McKibbin and White Sts. and go to your right on White.

- Turn left on Johnson Ave. On your right is the former Bushwick Terminal, which handled passenger service on the Long Island Rail Road until 1924 and to this day sees some freight traffic. The tower labeled VD 1858 is a brewery relic.

- Turn right on Bushwick Pl. One of the old breweries is on your right. It operated for about 100 years under different names, including Hittleman. For Brewers Row, turn left when you're in front of the playground, onto Meserole St. This and the next street, Scholes, were home in the late 1800s to 11 breweries from here to Lorimer St., six blocks on. Williamsburg's Brooklyn Brewery brought the biz back to the borough in 1996.

- Turn left on Bushwick Ave. Looking to the right down Montrose Ave., you can see the massive Gothic towers of Holy Trinity, a Catholic church from 1882. At Seigel St., the local library branch occupies a 100-year-old building that was originally an Andrew Carnegie library. The Hylan Houses next to the library took their name from John Hylan, who lived on Bushwick Ave. while he was mayor of NYC from 1918 to 1925. Hylan, a Brooklyn train engineer before he went into politics, railed against excessive corporate control, though he was backed by such overreaching potentates as Tammany Hall and William Randolph Hearst. As for corporate powers in Bushwick, Rheingold did its beer making on the seven-acre spread on your left that begins at Forrest St. and was the last Bushwick brewery to close. Now it's the Renaissance Estates and Rheingold Gardens, a suburban-type residential development with nearly a third of the units reserved for low-income households.

- At Arion Pl., make a 180-degree V turn to the right onto Beaver St. Turn left at Belvidere St., where the old Ulmer brewery on your right opened in 1872. The more visually interesting building is the storybook-like office next to it. The U embossed on its façade suggests it was part of the Ulmer operation.

- Turn left on Broadway. At Arion Pl., look for the WALL ST. etched on the building ahead of you. That was the original name of Arion; turn left to find out why it was changed . . .

- . . . because Arion Männerchor erected the most prominent structure on the block. Arion Männerchor was a German glee club—large and successful enough to build itself this red-brick palace on your left in 1887, complete with lyre designs in the balcony railings and corners of the roof (Arion is a lyre player in Greek mythology). The building later became a catering hall, then stood vacant and decaying for years. It was a fixer-upper when developers bought it and turned it into the Opera House Lofts. Longtime residents wary of gentrification sneered when the 66 apartments started renting out in late 2003, and it has been sprayed with graffiti on occasion.

- Turn right on Bushwick Ave., known in its high-falutin days as the Boulevard. A couple of blocks along on your right is St. Mark's, a preeminent church from Bushwick's days as a German community.

- Walk beneath the train at Myrtle Ave. Here commences the 1½-mile stretch where Bushwick's turn-of-the-century beer barons built their mansions. One of the most talked-about then and now is next to the KFC on your right. It belonged to William Ulmer, whose brewery we saw earlier, but is also identified with a subsequent owner, Dr. Frederick Cook, who had

*On Belvidere St.*

the juicier life story. Cook, the son of German immigrants, was on the medical team that accompanied Robert Peary's Arctic expeditions in the 1890s and was also an explorer in his own right. His claim of reaching the North Pole in April 1908—one year before Peary—could not be substantiated, and the ensuing investigation also discredited his earlier claim of being the first American to summit Mount McKinley. Peary went down in history as discoverer of the North Pole, but the legitimacy of Cook's claims is still being debated. Cook later served seven years in jail for stock fraud, but was eventually pardoned by FDR. As for Dr. Cook's former home, it had been abandoned for some time when it was purchased in 2000. The windows were restored in 2006, but the publicity-averse new owner has been silent about further renovation.

● Continue on Bushwick Ave. A block of old rowhouses in need of TLC is followed by a row that's been better cared for. After Hart St., old and new face off: the right side is modernized, the left a lovely row of wide bowfronts. At DeKalb Ave., the library on your right was built in 1905 in the Classical Revival tradition. Three blocks farther on Bushwick brings you to South Bushwick Reformed Church, which predates the beer-boom-funded construction of most of old Bushwick Ave. It has been here since 1853, built for a congregation founded in 1654. Many just call it the White Church, for obvious reasons.

● Turn left on Greene Ave. and right on Central Ave. and proceed to St. Barbara Roman Catholic Church, one of the tallest buildings in Brooklyn and possibly *the* most elaborate church in the city. Two towers, a polyhedral dome, tons of carvings—cherub faces and castles in the columns, expressive angels and saints above the doorway, horticultural designs all over. And there's more ornamentation inside! This Baroque fantasia was built in 1910 on the largesse of local brewer Leonard Eppig, who had a daughter named Barbara. Trot down Bleecker St. for a more thorough examination, but return to Central and walk toward Menahan St. The building next to the church is highly decorated in another way—with a mural painted over the entire front of El Puente, an organization for youth that conducts arts and educational programs promoting human rights and environmentalism.

● Turn right at Menahan. The Pentecostal church on your left is another formerly German house of worship.

- Turn left back onto Bushwick Ave., where two more churches built in the early years of the 20th century stand across from each other: Calvary & St. Cyprian's Episcopal and Mount of Olives Seventh Day Adventist. The next intersection has a splendid old mansion at almost every corner, beginning with the brick and granite castle on your near left. Across Grove St. is the real looker, tall and turreted. Opposite it geographically and stylistically is a solemn red-bricker, built three years before the others in 1887.

- At Linden St., the house on your left is a quirky compendium of half-moons and projections. From here you can see the towers of two more historic churches farther down Bushwick Ave.—United Methodist (originally Bushwick Avenue Central Methodist Episcopal Church) on the left and Bethesda Memorial Baptist (1896) on the right. Turn right on Linden.

- Turn right on Broadway, walking around a community garden with a grove of trees, to the J train.

## POINTS OF INTEREST

**Maria Hernandez Park** Irving Ave. between White and Starr Sts., Brooklyn, NY 11237
**Alex Aguinaga Restaurant** 214 Knickerbocker Ave., Brooklyn, NY 11237, 718-497-2828
**Justice Gilbert Ramirez Park** McKibbin and White Sts., Brooklyn, NY 11206

# route summary

1. Begin at Wyckoff and DeKalb Aves. and walk northwest on Wyckoff.

2. Turn left on Suydam St.

3. Enter Maria Hernandez Park at Irving Ave. Exit diagonally across at Starr St. and go right on Knickerbocker Ave.

4. Go left at Harrison Pl., right at Bogart St., and left at McKibbin St.

5. Turn right on White St.

6. Turn left on Johnson Ave.

7. Go right on Bushwick Pl., then left onto Meserole St.

8. Go left on Bushwick Ave.

9. Make a 180-degree turn to the right onto Beaver St., then a left on Belvidere St.

10. Turn left on Broadway and left on Arion Pl.

11. Turn right on Bushwick Ave.

12. Turn left at Greene Ave. and right at Central Ave.

13. Go right on Menahan.

14. Turn left back onto Bushwick Ave.

15. Go right on Linden St. and right on Broadway for the Gates Ave. subway station.

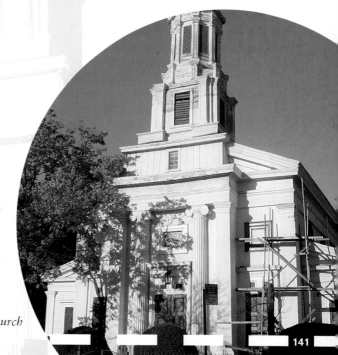

*South Bushwick Reformed Church*

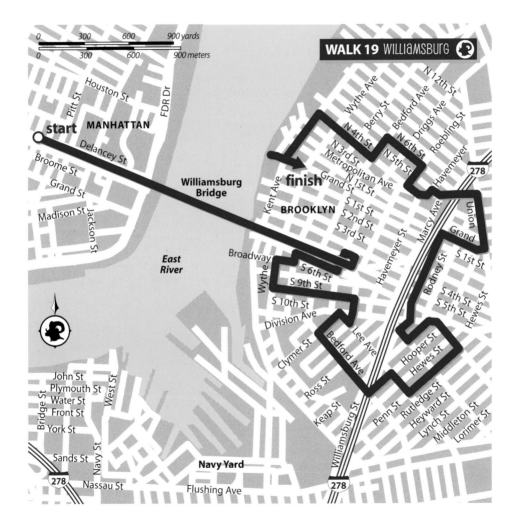

0 300 600 900 yards
0 300 600 900 meters

N 12th St
Wythe Ave
Berry St
Bedford Ave
Driggs Ave
N 4th St
Houston St
Pitt St
FDR Dr
N 3rd St
N 6th St
Roebling St
Havemeyer
MANHATTAN
start
Delancey St
Metropolitan Ave
N 5th St
278
Broome St
N 1st St
Grand St
finish
Grand St
Union
Grand
Grand St
Marcy Ave
Madison St
Jackson St
BROOKLYN
S 1st St
S 2nd St
S 1st St
Kent Ave
S 3rd St
Williamsburg
Bridge
Havemeyer St
East
River
Broadway
S 6th St
Rodney St
S 4th St
S 5th St
Wythe
S 9th St
Hewes St
S 10th St
Division Ave
Hooper St
Clymer St
Lee Ave
Hewes St
Bedford Ave
Ross St
Penn St
Rutledge St
Heyward St
Lynch St
Middleton St
Lorimer St
John St
Plymouth St
West St
Keap St
Water St
Bridge St
1st St
Front St
York St
Williamsburg St
Navy St
Sands St
278
Navy Yard
278
Nassau St
Flushing Ave

# 19 WILLIAMSBURG: HISTORIC, HASIDIC, HISPANIC, AND HOT!

**BOUNDARIES:** Essex St. (Manhattan), Bedford Ave., Penn St., Metropolitan Ave. or N. 6th St.
**DISTANCE:** Approx. 4½ or 5¾ miles, depending on route chosen
**SUBWAY:** F to Delancey St.

Williamsburg's 21st-century reinvention as hipster haven Billyburg occurred after decades of poverty and neglect. It's only the latest transformation for an area that's had many identities. From a farming village within the 17th-century Dutch settlement of Boswijck (Bushwick), Williamsburg grew into a center of brewing and manufacturing and by 1852 was large enough to charter as a city. It lost its independence, and the *h* at the end of its name, when annexed by the city of Brooklyn three years later. Its days as a well-off suburb and resort came to an end with the 1903 opening of the Williamsburg Bridge, which you cross on this walk. Immigrants crowded out of Manhattan's Lower East Side, directly across the river, began to fill tenements in Williamsburg—an era depicted in the coming-of-age novel *A Tree Grows in Brooklyn*. New immigrant communities arose after World War II: first Hasidic Jews from Eastern Europe and later Puerto Ricans and other Hispanics. Both groups reside in what's known as the Southside, or Los Sures to Latinos. In the 1990s, artists who couldn't afford the East Village discovered the Northside. That paved the way for an influx of white middle-class college grads with bohemian aspirations. Vaulted to the forefront of Brooklyn's renaissance, Williamsburg may yet be made over by developers of luxury residential properties.

● Begin on Manhattan's Lower East Side. From the subway, walk on Delancey St. toward the bridge and cross to the pedestrian lane at Clinton St. Follow it onto the north walkway (to your left) of the bridge. The Williamsburg was the first East River span built after the Brooklyn Bridge, supplanting it (by five feet) as the world's longest suspension bridge and establishing steel as the preferred material for bridges. For pedestrians, a couple of things differ on the Williamsburg compared to the Manhattan and Brooklyn bridges. The Williamsburg is farthest north, so it provides a closer view of Midtown Manhattan. Because the East River curves almost 90 degrees below the Williamsburg, you see less of Lower Manhattan and more of Brooklyn from this bridge—Downtown, Dumbo, the Navy Yard, and, of course, the borough's tallest building, the Williamsburgh Savings Bank tower. The lone skyscraper to your left as you near the Brooklyn side is Queens' tallest building, Citibank.

● As you descend the bridge toward Williamsburg, the old Domino Sugar factory dominates the shoreline to your left. Brooklyn was the sugar-refining capital of the United States from the late 19th century through most of the 20th. Now a battle over the Domino site's future is under way. The new owners reportedly plan to build four residential towers, but community groups want it granted landmark status and other government and citizen interests are hankering to adapt it for recreational and cultural uses.

● One more distinction of the Williamsburg Bridge: It provides the best-looking entree into Brooklyn, courtesy of Continental Army Plaza and the Williamsburg Trust Company. Cross the street to your left as you step off the bridge, bringing you in front of the gorgeous Neoclassic building erected by the bank in 1906. Cross S. 5th Pl. to the plaza, with a statue of George Washington during the arduous wintertime campaign at Valley Forge. The sculptor chose not to glorify triumph in war, but to honor a warrior's fortitude. Wander around the plaza, which used to be a major trolley hub, then go back across S. 5th Pl. and down S. 5th St.

● Turn left on Driggs Ave. and walk under the bridge to Broadway. This was the central business district when Williamsburg was its own city. Some of it resembles Manhattan's Soho, with such cast-iron edifices as the former shoe warehouse (built in 1882) on your left. On your right is another domed gem, erected in 1875. Now a branch of HSBC, it served as Williamsburgh Savings Bank's flagship until the clock-tower building went up in Fort Greene in 1929. If possible, go inside, where WSB is etched in glass panes around the base of the 110-foot dome. Then cross Broadway to another famous Williamsburg destination, Peter Luger. It originated in 1876 as a billiards cafe and bowling alley and in 1887 became a restaurant that served porterhouse steak and only porterhouse steak—not even any veggies on the side. The menu diversified in 1947, though porterhouse remains its raison d'être. Luger is considered the best steakhouse in the city, maybe even the country or, according to one-time customer Alfred Hitchcock, "the universe."

- Turn right on Broadway, admiring the craftsmanship on the 19th-century buildings as you proceed toward Bedford Ave. Another former bank, #135 on your right at Bedford, was built in French Second Empire style in 1868 and now houses the Williamsburg Art & Historical Center, a pioneering proponent of the local arts scene. There are at least 35 art galleries in Williamsburg, most of them north of the bridge.

- Cross Bedford and walk down S. 6th St. to your right. The weathered building on your right with a top floor of arched windows above façade medallions was built for the legitimate stage in 1891 but became a burlesque house.

- Turn left on Berry St. and right on Broadway. If you want something to eat, on your right are Diner, a restaurant in a 1920s Kullman car, and Marlow & Sons, a raw-bar, bistro and bakery. Farther down on your left, luxury condos in the former Gretsch musical-instrument factory sold out quickly (rapper Busta Rhymes and actress Annabella Sciorra were among the buyers) amid protests from Hasidim about its proximity to their community.

- Go left on Wythe Ave., then left on S. 9th, a street that's been a heart of Latino Williamsburg but has gained a Hasidic presence. The playground at Bedford, with animal sculptings on its gate and pigeon-shooing iron owls on its lampposts, is tied up in the history of Schaefer beer. The brewery traded this parcel to the city in the 1950s for a former ferry landing five blocks away—an acquisition that allowed Schaefer (the last Brooklyn brewery to close, in 1976) to expand its waterfront plant. Continuing on S. 9th St., cross Driggs to the landmark New England Congregational Church, built in 1853. The materials and style broke with

*Williamsburg Bridge*

the Congregationalist tradition of a white exterior and spire. The church became a Spanish-speaking Pentecostal house, La Luz del Mundo, in 1955.

● Turn right on Roebling St., right on Lee Ave., and left on Clymer St. Go left on Bedford, a moneyed street at the turn of the century. Jewish youth now attend school in mansions where the upper crust of Wasp society used to gather. The Congress Club met in #505 (built in 1896), the Hanover Club at #563 (1875).

● Cross over the Brooklyn-Queens Expressway (BQE) and turn left on Hooper St. Then make a right on Lee, the Hasids' busiest shopping street (deserted on Saturday, when stores are closed for the Sabbath). All these streets you've passed or walked on since turning onto Bedford were named after signers of the Declaration of Independence. Williamsburg has 27 such streets in all.

● Turn left on Penn St. Walk two lovely blocks to Harrison St. and turn left. After Hooper, Harrison merges into Division Ave. Go one more block and turn left onto Keap St. (town planners misread Thomas McKean's signature on the Declaration of Independence as Thomas M. Keap). On your left after turning from Division is the second-oldest synagogue in Brooklyn, built in 1876 and now used as a Hasidic school. Farther down the block on your right, another Hasidic school occupies the old Eastern District High School, whose alumni include Mel Brooks, Barry Manilow, and Henry Miller.

● Make a right on Marcy Ave. and look up as you're walking on this block to fully appreciate the extravagant architecture of Eastern District H.S.

● Turn right on Rodney St. At the next corner on your left, the local branch of the Brooklyn Public Library sits like an open book on a triangular plot facing the BQE. It's old but not old enough to explain the Williamsburgh spelling. When the library was built in 1905—one of Andrew Carnegie's first library endowments in Brooklyn—Williamsburg had been without its *h* for several decades. Continue on Rodney, which takes you from S. 9th to S. 5th St. in a single block. The playground to your left was the neighborhood's compensation for having a highway sliced through it.

- Turn right on Grand St., where you can visit the Photo Gallery of Williamsburg at #437. Past Keap, Grand leads into Borinquen Pl. (an extension of Grand). Go one more block and turn left on Union Ave. On your right between Powers and Ainslie Sts., check out the bottle-cap mosaic on the wall outside Barcade. The bar inside this converted garage features some two dozen microbrews on tap and about that many 1980s-era arcade games.

- If you wish to stop at this point, there's an L/G subway station at Metropolitan Ave. Or continue through more of hipster Williamsburg and to the waterfront.

Addendum:

- Turn left on Metropolitan. On your right, benches surround Macri Triangle, a little park containing a bocce court and a World War II memorial full of Italian surnames. Italians started settling in the neighborhood for the factory work 100 or so years ago. Every July, Williamsburg's Italians still celebrate the Feast of the Giglio, during which hundreds of men carry an 85-foot, 2-ton statue of a saint through the streets, accompanied by a brass band.

- Walk on Metropolitan and go right onto N. 5th St. beneath the very tall Roman Catholic Church of the Annunciation. It was constructed in 1869 and joined 20 years later by its convent across Havemeyer St., an attractive building that's been converted to condominiums.

- Turn left on Havemeyer and right back onto Metropolitan. Across the avenue, the unique storefront museum called the City Reliquary displays NYC memorabilia and artifacts including Statue of Liberty souvenirs, parts of old subway cars, masonry and metal pieces from landmarks, and a geology exhibit of rock and soil samples taken around the five boroughs.

- From Metropolitan, take N. 4th St. to your right, then turn right on Roebling. Oslo Coffee Company, on your right, roasts and grinds their own beans and makes espresso drinks rivaling those in Italy (according to devotees).

- Turn left on N. 6th St. and then left at Bedford, the central thoroughfare of hipster Williamsburg. On your right at N. 5th, the former Realform Girdle factory was one of the first industrial conversions. The ground floor contains a communal living room, with seating, computers, and reading material, plus a mini-mall of shops, including Spoonbill & Sugartown Booksellers.

● Turn right on N. 4th and proceed to Kent Ave., where you'll be in front of the first of three high-rises planned for the sprawling Northside Piers residential complex. Turn left on Kent, a ghost town not long ago but now among the hottest real estate in NYC. Preservationists have been trying to rein in development, while others are concerned there won't be enough waterfront left for a public park. The white building at the corner of N. 3rd—once a warehouse for wholesale grocer Austin, Nichols & Company—has been especially contentious, with its fate yo-yoing since 2005: the landmarks commission granted it landmark status, a decision that was revoked by the city council, whose vote was then vetoed by the mayor, who was then overruled by the city council. Though aesthetically unremarkable, the 1915 monolith is noteworthy for its architect: Cass Gilbert designed it around the same time he was working on the venerable Woolworth Building in Lower Manhattan.

● Turn right when you see the first Domino Sugar building, at Grand St., and wrap up the walk at Grand Ferry Park, the only patch of Williamsburg waterfront currently available to the public. Certainly views like this merit a more spacious milieu from which to enjoy them. Read the history of the site on the smokestack left behind by Pfizer; if you're wondering why the pharmaceutical giant was mixing molasses here, it contributed to penicillin production.

● Walk up Grand to Wythe Ave. and take the Q59 bus to the Metropolitan Ave./Lorimer St. station of the L/G trains.

*Originally, Williamsburgh Savings Bank*

## POINTS OF INTEREST

**Williamsburg Trust Company** S. 5th St. and S. 5th Pl., Brooklyn, NY 11211

**Williamsburgh Savings Bank (HSBC)** 175 Broadway, Brooklyn, NY 11211

**Peter Luger** 178 Broadway, Brooklyn, NY 11211, 718-387-7400

**Williamsburg Art & Historical Center** 135 Broadway, Brooklyn, NY 11211, 718-486-7372

**Diner** 85 Broadway, Brooklyn, NY 11211, 718-486-3077

**Marlow & Sons** 81 Broadway, Brooklyn, NY 11211, 718-384-1441

**Brooklyn Public Library–Williamsburgh** Division and Marcy Aves., Brooklyn, NY 11211, 718-302-3485

**Photo Gallery of Williamsburg** 437 Grand St., Brooklyn, NY 11211, 718-782-3433

**Barcade** 388 Union Ave., Brooklyn, NY 11211, 718-302-6464

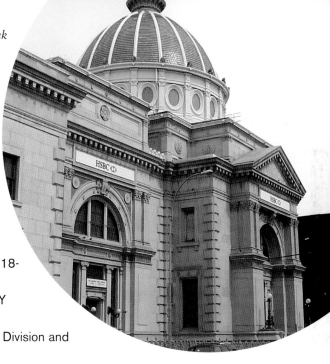

## ADDENDUM

**City Reliquary** 370 Metropolitan Ave., Brooklyn, NY 11211, 718-782-4842

**Oslo Coffee Company** 133 Roebling St., Brooklyn, NY 11211, 718-782-0332

**Spoonbill & Sugartown Booksellers** 218 Bedford Ave., Brooklyn, NY 12111, 718-387-7322

**Grand Ferry Park** Grand St. off Kent Ave., Brooklyn, NY 11211

# route summary

1. Begin on the Manhattan side of the Williamsburg Bridge.
2. Cross the bridge and proceed into Continental Army Plaza on your left.
3. Cross S. 5th Pl. and walk down S. 5th St.
4. Turn left on Driggs Ave.
5. Turn right onto Broadway.
6. Go to your right down S. 6th St.
7. Turn left at Berry St. and right on Broadway.
8. Go left on Wythe Ave., then left on S. 9th St.
9. In quick succession, go right on Roebling St., right on Lee Ave., and left on Clymer St. to reach Bedford, where you turn left.
10. Go left on Hooper St., then right on Lee.
11. Turn left on Penn St.
12. Turn left on Harrison St., which merges into Division Ave. Turn left on Keap St. from Division.
13. Turn right on Marcy Ave.
14. Turn right on Rodney St.
15. Turn right on Grand St. and stay on it for the Borinquen Pl. extension. Then turn left on Union Ave.
16. Get the L or G train at Union and Metropolitan Aves.

# addendum

17. Turn left on Metropolitan.
18. Turn right on N. 5th St.
19. Turn left on Havemeyer St. and right back onto Metropolitan.
20. Go right on N. 4th St. and right on Roebling.
21. Turn left on N. 6th St., then left on Bedford.
22. Turn right on N. 4th. and left on Kent Ave.
23. Turn right on Grand St.
24. Walk east on Grand to Wythe Ave. for the Q59 bus to the L/G trains.

*Grand Ferry Park*

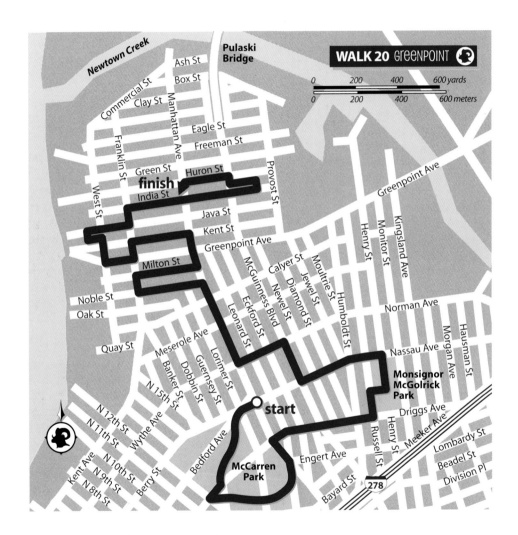

Newtown Creek

Pulaski Bridge

**WALK 20** GREENPOINT

0    200    400    600 yards
0    200    400    600 meters

Ash St
Box St
Commercial St
Clay St
Manhattan Ave
Franklin Ave
Eagle St
Freeman St
West St
Green St
Huron St
**finish**
India St
Provost St
Greenpoint Ave
Java St
Kent St
Greenpoint Ave
Henry St
Monitor St
Kingsland Ave
Milton St
McGuinness Blvd
Calyer St
Moultrie St
Humboldt St
Noble St
Newel St
Jewel St
Diamond St
Norman Ave
Oak St
Eckford St
Leonard St
Quay St
Meserole Ave
Lorimer St
Nassau Ave
Morgan Ave
Hausman St
Banker St
Dobbin St
Guernsey St
**Monsignor McGolrick Park**
N 15th St
Driggs Ave
Wythe Ave
○ **start**
Henry St
Meeker Ave
N 12th St
N 11th St
Bedford Ave
Lombardy St
Kent Ave
N 10th St
Russell St
Beadel St
N 9th St
Berry St
**McCarren Park**
Engert Ave
Division Pl
N 8th St
Bayard St
278

# 20 Greenpoint: Industrial Center With a Polish Flavor

BOUNDARIES: **Huron St., Russell St., Bayard St., West St.**
DISTANCE: **Approx. 3¾ miles**
SUBWAY: **G to Nassau Ave.**

Greenpoint was one of Brooklyn's centers of the "black arts," with more than 50 oil refineries and 20 glass factories in operation in the late 19th century. But industry was on the decline by the mid-20th century, and its vestigial infrastructure today marks Greenpoint as a neighborhood of contrasts, sometimes on the same street. Some abandoned factories and riverfront street ends are given over to litter and graffiti, while other old buildings have been cleaned up and repurposed for artist studios, new businesses, and desirable apartments. Further improvements to the housing stock and outdoor spaces are expected as the hipster/artist spillover from neighboring Williamsburg continues. Meanwhile, Greenpoint's most steadfast identity has been as a Little Poland. Poles first moved here during the huge influx of Eastern European immigration in the late 19th century, and later generations fled Nazism, then communism, and then the post-communist uncertainty. The neighborhood was still receiving thousands of new Polish residents a year in the 1990s.

● Walk west from Manhattan and Nassau Aves. on Nassau. Just past Lorimer St., where Nassau and Bedford Aves. cross, is Father Jerzy Popieluszko Square, perhaps the most sacred of several tributes to Polish heroes. The murdered anticommunist priest is honored with a granite bust and a garden of colorful flowers. Be sure to find the smaller sculpture of outstretched arms—symbolizing the yearning for freedom and peace—on the other side of the flagpole in the square; it can get obscured by foliage.

● Cross Bedford to McCarren Park, a 35-acre green space that sprawls across five blocks and demarcates Greenpoint from Williamsburg (both neighborhoods claim the park). Enter at Lorimer and Bedford and take the path to your left. Go to the right when the path diverges, then exit via the second path on your left, at Driggs Ave. and N. 12th St. Cross the street to the Russian Orthodox Cathedral of the Transfiguration of Our Lord, which was built around 1920 and purportedly modeled after the czar's

Winter Palace in St. Petersburg; if you can get inside you'll see icons painted by monks in Kiev.

- Go back into McCarren Park across N. 12th from the church and take a stroll through Green Dome Garden on your right.

- Cross Union Ave. and walk east through the park or along Bayard St., its southern border. As you approach Lorimer, there's another community garden (on your right if you're in the park, on your left if you're on Bayard)—smaller and much less formal than Green Dome.

- Cross Lorimer and take a look, through the overgrowth and gate, at what used to be a favorite gathering place for the people of Greenpoint and surrounding neighborhoods. The McCarren pool was the largest (capacity: 6,800) of 11 public swimming pools constructed in New York City during the Depression by the Works Progress Administration. Once compared to the Roman baths at Caracalla, it began to fall into disrepair in the 1970s and closed in 1984. Residents have revived it in recent years as a performance and event space.

- Follow the path around the pool to Leonard St. and continue walking beside the park, past basketball courts on your left.

- Go to the right on Driggs. Between Leonard and Eckford Sts., the building with reddish-brown trim on your right is the Polish National Home, a cultural center that has kept the homeland's heritage alive for immigrants and their American-born children. It now houses Warsaw, a popular nightspot.

- Continuing on Driggs, you'll come to Father Studzinski Square, a not always well-maintained patch between Graham Ave. and McGuinness Blvd. that honors a long-time pastor of Greenpoint's major Polish church, St. Stanislaus. Reach the church by proceeding on Driggs to Humboldt St. Affectionately called St. Stans, the commanding St. Stanislaus Kostka Vincentian Fathers Church has stood here since the 1890s. Street signs outside the church commemorate visits by Lech Walesa and Pope John Paul II. The marble interior is worth seeing.

- Go one more block on Driggs and turn left on Russell St. Across the street from the Lutheran Church of the Messiah is pleasant Monsignor McGolrick Park. The entry gates on Russell are flanked by munching-squirrel statuettes. At the center of the park is the colonnaded shelter pavilion, built in 1910 and listed on the National Register of Historic Places. There's an angel statue in memory of World War I vets and a larger monument on the east side in honor of the USS *Monitor,* the Civil War ship built at Greenpoint's Continental Iron Works.

- Leave the park at the corner of Russell and Nassau and walk to your left on Nassau. One of the best Polish restaurants in the neighborhood is on your left at Humboldt: Old Poland. For a sampling of favorites, try the bargain-priced combination plate of potato pancakes, pierogies, kielbasa, stuffed cabbage, and bigos (a sauerkraut and beef stew). There are more Polish restaurants elsewhere on Nassau and on Manhattan, and almost all are inexpensive and casual. Or stop in at a deli, where you can mix and match dishes sold by the pound or piece, then top off the meal with some babka or a big jelly dough-nut from one of the many bakeries. As you continue on Nassau, and later on Manhattan, you'll notice plenty of other Polish businesses—butchers, law offices, spas, and psychics—as well as coffeehouses and yoga studios that serve the new, young residents of Greenpoint. You might enjoy exploring in the Polish drugstores, which stock a lot of herbs and holistic-type products.

- Go right on McGuinness Blvd. On the right is the new headquarters of the Polish & Slavic Federal Credit Union, a financial bedrock of the community for several decades. The façade depicts coats of arms of various cities in Poland—the mermaid, for instance, is a symbol of Warsaw.

*In Monsignor McGolrick Park*

- Turn left on Norman Ave. and then right on Manhattan Ave., where you'll find remnants of days gone by mixing with the new. At #723–725, two eras are represented: The Eckerd drugstore owes its temple-esque façade to the building's original existence as a 1920s theater, while the ramp, oval floor, and disco ball (!) inside remain from when it was a roller rink. Next door, Peter Pan Donut & Pastry Shop has been serving up plump, moist homemade doughnuts for over 50 years. You may put on weight just examining their alluringly gluttonous varieties (apple crumb is a specialty). Meanwhile, the turn-of-the-century sidewalk clock in front of #733 and curved cast-iron street lamps along Manhattan hark back to a more distant age. These and other iron objects are a source of local pride, as ironworking was a big business in Greenpoint. At #765, look up at the flourishy upper level and its billboards for Europa Night Club. This disco, whose entrance is around the corner on Meserole Ave., attracts young Polish-Americans and contains an art gallery that hosts exhibitions as well as music, dance, and poetry performances on Art Nights. The club is known in Europe, so some Polish immigrants and visitors make it their first stop for socializing when they get to New York. At the corner of Manhattan Ave. and Calyer St. is a reminder of the days when bank architecture was majestic. This 1908 Pantheon simulacrum was the main office of the Green Point Savings Bank, but is now just one branch of that bank (now called the North Fork Bank). Don't miss its beautiful marble interior.

- Turn left on Noble St. and instantaneously the bustle of Manhattan Ave. is silenced. On your right, the Polish National Alliance, or Zjednoczenie Polsko Narodowe—see the ZPN imprinted in the stoop—is a longstanding fraternal and social-services organization. As opposed to this still-vital institution, two houses of worship on the block have been vacated: Union Baptist Church, built in 1863, which is right next to ZPN; and the Ahawath Israel synagogue (1904), farther down on the left. Also on the left is an Italianate group at #128–#132 from 1867. During Greenpoint's industrial boom, factory owners and managers lived in the refined brick homes on Noble and other side streets, whereas workers inhabited the less distinguished housing in the area.

- Just as the ambience altered sharply when you turned from Manhattan onto Noble, look across Franklin St. for another drastic contrast. Noble transforms not only from residential to industrial but also from pretty to eyesore-ish.

- Turn right on Franklin and then right on Milton St., heading back toward Manhattan Ave. Here, as on the other alphabetically named streets off Manhattan, you see a dichotomy common in Greenpoint: mundane aluminum-sided rowhouses near elegant brownstones and brick homes. The detached mini-mansion at #136, now a Reformed church, was the home of Thomas Smith, who helped bring the European art (and business) of porcelain making to the United States with his Greenpoint-based Union Porcelain Works. On your right, St. John's Lutheran Church was built in 1892 for a parish of German immigrants and has Bavarian woodworking on its interior walls.

- The St. John's spire rises across from that of St. Anthony of Padua/St. Alphonsius, on Manhattan Ave. at Milton. This handsomely adorned church (built in 1874) reflects fluctuations in local demographics: the two congregations that occupy it originally served Irish and German residents, respectively, but dwindling memberships eventually led to a merger, and the combined congregation now comprises mostly Poles and Latinos. Facing the church, go to your left on Manhattan.

- When you reach Kent St., the tan building with a step-shape front down the street to your right is the Polish & Slavic Culture Center, a social hub of the community founded by the same clergyman who established the credit union. But you want to go left on Kent for more historic homes and houses of worship. Just past Manhattan on your right is St. Elias Byzantine Catholic Church, a Dutch Reformed church when it opened in 1870. The oldest church in Greenpoint is midway down the block: the Episcopal Church of the Ascension, built in 1865. This block of Kent also contains probably the oldest homes in the neighborhood, dating to the mid-19th century. The house at #130 was the residence of steamship builder Neziah Bliss, recognized as a founder of Greenpoint because he was one of the first industrialists to buy land here.

- Turn left at Franklin. On your left at the next corner are the offices of the Polish daily newspaper *Nowy Dziennik*. They occupy an 1895 Renaissance Revival building, with terra cotta frieze, that originally housed a bank and later the Polish Home Service.

- Cross Franklin and walk to 61 Greenpoint Ave., the factory where a math teacher's best friend, the Eberhard Faber pencil, was manufactured from 1872 until the company relocated in 1956. Sharpened pencils are part of the building's facade, as is the star-in-diamond trademark of Eberhard Faber's Mongol pencils.

- Turn right on West St., then go left on Java St. to the water's edge to get an idea of Greenpoint's potential for redevelopment. The great view of Midtown Manhattan and the Williamsburg Bridge from Greenpoint has the city and developers talking about a riverside esplanade and recreational areas. While some spots haven't been renewed much at all, as you head back east on Java you can see that businesses and studios are already occupying some of the old warehouse space.

- Turn left when you're back at Franklin. The Astral, a red-brick apartment building on the east side of the street, has been granted city landmark status. Built in 1886 for employees of Charles Pratt's Astral Oil, the Romanesque Revival building was an upgrade from the then-typical homely, crowded worker housing. And unlike those tenements, it had indoor plumbing and hot water.

- At India St., turn right and proceed past Manhattan Ave. and then McGuinness Blvd. Here, one aspect of Greenpoint's past—metalworking—stays alive, employing young artists and thriving as an economic concern. If you pop in at 220 India St., owner Paige Tooker will be glad to show you around the New Foundry, which casts sculptures and statues. More industrial-type casting is done at Bedi-Makky Foundry across the street. It was here, when the operation was named Bedi-Rassy, that the Iwo Jima monument was cast—that iconic image of World War II troops raising the U.S. flag in the Pacific.

- Go back to McGuinness and turn right. At Huron St., look to your right: those futuristic domes are part of a water-treatment plant for Newtown Creek, which separates Brooklyn from Queens to the near north and east. In Greenpoint's industrial heyday it was as busy a commercial waterway as the Mississippi River, and these days it's being eyed for possible recreational development. Two of the bridges across the creek are named for Polish generals who fought on the colonists' side in the American Revolution: the Pulaski Bridge, which you see ahead of you extending from McGuinness Blvd., and the Kosciuszko, part of the Brooklyn-Queens Expressway.

- Turn left on Huron and get the G train at Manhattan and India.

## POINTS OF INTEREST

**Father Jerzy Popieluszko Square** Bedford and Nassau Aves., Brooklyn, NY 11222

**McCarren Park** Bedford Ave. and Bayard St., Brooklyn, NY 11222

**Green Dome Garden** McCarren Park at N. 12th St., Brooklyn, NY 11222

**Warsaw** Polish National Home, 261 Driggs Ave., Brooklyn, NY 11222, 718-387-0505

**Monsignor McGolrick Park** Driggs Ave. and Russell St., Brooklyn, NY 11222

**Old Poland** 190 Nassau Ave., Brooklyn, NY 11222, 718-349-7775

**Peter Pan Donut & Pastry Shop** 727 Manhattan Ave., Brooklyn, NY 11222, 718-383-9442

**Europa Night Club** 98 Meserole Ave., Brooklyn, NY 11222, 718-383-5723

**Green Point Savings Bank (North Fork Bank)** 807 Manhattan Ave., Brooklyn, NY 11222, 718-706-2901

**New Foundry New York** 220 India St., Brooklyn, NY 11222, 718-389-8172

## route summary

1. Begin at Manhattan and Nassau Aves. and head west on Nassau.
2. Cross Bedford Ave. and walk through McCarren Park to Driggs Ave. and N. 12th St.
3. Walk through (or on the outskirts of) McCarren Park to Leonard St.
4. Walk north along the park.
5. Turn right on Driggs.
6. Turn left on Russell St. and enter Monsignor McGolrick Park.
7. Exit the park on Nassau and go left.
8. Turn right on McGuinness Blvd.
9. Turn left on Norman Ave. and right on Manhattan.
10. Turn left on Noble St.
11. Turn right on Franklin St. and right on Milton St.
12. Turn left on Manhattan and left on Kent St.
13. Turn left on Franklin, right on Greenpoint Ave., and right on West St.
14. Turn left on Java St. to reach the river.
15. Walk away from the river on Java and turn left on Franklin, then right on India St.
16. After reaching 220 India St., return to McGuinness Blvd. and turn right.
17. Turn left on Huron St. and get the subway at Manhattan and India.

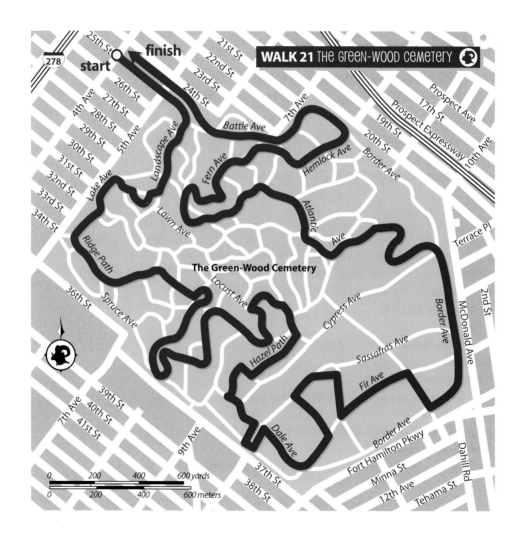

**The Green-Wood Cemetery**

start

finish

278

25th St
21st St
22nd St
23rd St
24th St
26th St
27th St
28th St
29th St
30th St
31st St
32nd St
33rd St
34th St
4th Ave
5th Ave
Landscape Ave
Lake Ave
Fern Ave
Battle Ave
7th Ave
Hemlock Ave
19th St
20th St
17th St
Prospect Ave
Prospect Expressway
Border Ave
10th Ave
Lawn Ave
Atlantic Ave
Terrace Pl
Ridge Path
36th St
Spruce Ave
Locust Ave
Cypress Ave
Border Ave
McDonald Ave
2nd St
7th Ave
39th St
40th St
41st St
Hazel Path
Sassafras Ave
Fir Ave
9th Ave
Dale Ave
37th St
38th St
Border Ave
Fort Hamilton Pkwy
Minna St
12th Ave
Tehama St
Dahill Rd

0   200   400   600 yards
0   200   400   600 meters

# 21 THE GREEN-WOOD CEMETERY: GARDEN OASIS FOR ETERNAL REPOSE

BOUNDARIES: **4th Ave., 20th St., Fort Hamilton Pkwy., 36th St. (all outside the cemetery)**
DISTANCE: **Approx. 4½ miles**
SUBWAY: **R to 25th St.**

Yes, the "The" belongs in the name, as does the hyphen, though Green and Wood are not the cemetery's patrons, but two pastoral images from this 478-acre greensward of hills and ponds and a fascinating collection of statuary. About 560,000 people have been laid to rest here since the first burial in September 1840. They include prominent players in Brooklyn's growth as a city; people central to the civic, religious, and cultural history of NYC; and artists and inventors known the world over. But focusing strictly on the deceased is missing the point, and beauty, of Green-Wood, one of the nation's first cemeteries not located within a churchyard. It was designed to be a rural oasis in a harsh industrialized city, a place to reconnect with nature and reflect on life and death in a calm, attractive setting. It was a quintessentially Victorian concept, glorifying death in such an aesthetic manner. The ideals of the age are also represented in other ways, from recurring imagery in the monuments—a sphere to symbolize eternity, for instance—to the personal and often dramatic flourishes on gravesites, to the euphemistic language of the epitaphs, in which the deceased "left his earthly labors" or "had issue" (i.e., children). For most of the 20th century, admission was limited to lot owners, but now the cemetery is open daily to visitors, with extended hours in summer. Such openness restores Green-Wood's stature as a park destination: in the mid-1800s, it was second only to Niagara Falls in drawing tourists.

● **From the subway, walk up 25th St. to 5th Ave. Before crossing 5th to the cemetery entrance, note the florists on your right. Their building, not currently in the best shape, is listed on the National Register of Historic Places as the Weir Greenhouse, its name upon opening in 1895. It once had a grandeur befitting Green-Wood. The monument company behind it on 25th has served the cemetery even longer—since 1854. Its oeuvre includes the Green-Wood graves of Horace Greeley, Peter Cooper, and Nathaniel Currier.**

● Cross the avenue and enter through Richard Upjohn's Gothic gates. These were created in 1861, after the cemetery had become a success, and feature sandstone bas-reliefs of death and resurrection. You may hear squawking coming from the gates or see birds flying in and out of the peaks. These are green parakeets from South America that started nesting here after they broke out of their crate at the airport in 1980. Or so the story goes.

● Through the main gate, turn right on Landscape Ave. and walk toward the chapel. Pass an old hitching post on your right from the horse-drawn carriage days. Opposite the flower bed in front of the chapel, a little angel marks the resting place of a brother and sister who died within a year of each other, a sweet but sad monument typical of children's graves at Green-Wood. Behind this plot is a grave topped by a draped urn, another recurring sight. It symbolizes what is left on earth after the soul ascends to heaven: the body, or container of the soul (represented by the urn), and the cover of the casket (the shroud). The chapel itself, modeled on Christ Church in Oxford, England, was designed by the architects of Grand Central Terminal. It's open to the public when no services are being conducted inside and also hosts lectures and theatrical performances, almost always with a Green-Wood interee as the subject matter.

● With your back to the chapel, go left up the ramp to Landscape Ave., where you can see a strangely sensual male angel, large wings rising high above his head. Turn left on Landscape. At Valley Ave., you'll pass a tall angel with raised arm towering over the Siefke family plot, which blooms with roses in season. Continue on Landscape and turn left on Ridge Path. Past a large tree on your right, next to the Nash obelisk, the lamb sculpture at the Hickson grave is eroding. Lambs are a common motif on children's graves, symbolizing their innocence. Go onto the grass to your left from the path and walk past two crosses to the Tiffany graves. Charles Lewis Tiffany founded the jewelry store that bears his name; his son Louis Comfort was the stained-glass artist who made windows and lamps. The N.A. after Louis's names on his wives' graves refers to his membership in the National Academy of Design.

● Go down Vale Path next to the Tiffany graves and turn left on Valley Ave. As you walk along Valley beside the water, you should see a statue of a woman holding a book and raising an arm. The grave is marked I.O.O.F. for the International Order of Odd Fellows, a charitable organization founded in 17th-century England when it was odd for people to join a group to help others. Turn left at Dew Path, then right on Hillside Path. Asher Durand, Hudson River School painter, is buried on your left behind the Woodmans, his daughter's in-laws. Durand's masterpiece, *Kindred Spirits,* sold in 2005 for $35 million, a record for an American painting. Follow Hillside to the right back to Valley, where you can't miss the ornate tomb of John Matthews on your left. Matthews, known as the soda-fountain king for his invention of machines that carbonated and dispensed beverages, is the man laying and looking up at a ceiling that depicts events in his life. The seated figure above symbolizes grief. Some of the human faces carved on the structure are his family members.

- Walk downhill on Walnut Ave. and go left at Lake Ave. On your left, a woman with flowers stands over the grave of George Tilyou, the Coney Island legend who created its great amusement park, Steeplechase.

- Continue on Lake Ave. past the grove of bushes on your right. Turn right on Sylvan Ave. and look for three interesting graves in the island on your left: George W. Struthers, who was reinterred five years after his death when fellow soldiers learned his body had not been claimed; Do-Hum-Me, a Sac Indian chief's daughter who became a star attraction of P.T. Barnum shows; and Rocco Agoglia, with a domed tomb and defiant angel sitting guard.

- Proceed on Sylvan Ave. past Sylvan Water on your left. Just before the next fork, find D.R. Bennett's grave, embossed with a literal interpretation of the adage "the pen is mightier than the sword." Bennett, a Shaker turned freethinker, was jailed for mailing out his antireligion tracts—deemed obscene under the Comstock laws that prevented such material from

*The main gates of Green-Wood*

being sent through the mail. As you can tell from his verbose grave, he couldn't have been an easy person to muzzle.

- Turn left on Spruce Ave. Then go left on Anemone Path and right on Ridge Path. Stay to the right when the path diverges. One of the tombs along the pond that you're overlooking contains songwriter Fred Ebb, who penned the lyrics to *Cabaret, Chicago,* and "New York, New York."

- Go left onto Cedar Path, then left on Lake Ave. Take Ravine Path on your right up and over to Oak Ave., where you go left. Crusading newspaperman Horace Greeley is buried on a hill to your left. Despite his oft-quoted advice, the bust of him does not face west. You can spot it from the avenue, but you'll have to climb if you want to see the bas-relief images of his profession (man at printing press, quill pen and paper, etc.).

- Across Oak Ave. from Greeley's grave, follow Winterberry Path to a big, knobby tree. Go left to the angel of death (sans left hand) weeping over the Cassard grave. The wife's family, Platt, has graves nearby with much floral ornamentation. Several 9/11 victims are buried in this area, including firefighters Cherry, Agnello, and Vega in a cluster directly across from Greeley and a couple of more groupings as you continue across the grass. Green-Wood contains the graves of about 75 people who died in the terrorist attacks.

- With your back to Greeley's grave, go down the lawn to Landscape Ave. and go right. Turn left on Circling Path, then take the path to the right of the tree. Between two tall trees on your right, there's a statue of a man with a doting young woman—the GRAND-PA AND HIS LOVING GRANDDAUGHTER who are buried together.

- Go back on Circling Path and continue in the direction you had been headed. Turn left when you reach the avenue. As it curves around, you'll find the largest mausoleum in Green-Wood, created in the 1870s for the Steinways, piano makers extraordinaire, by John Moffitt, sculptor of the bas-reliefs on the entrance gates. It cost almost $2 million in today's dollars and contains 119 rooms, with space for as many as 200 interees, though fewer than 60 Steinways ended up here. Continue around the oval to Thorn Path and go left. Cross Highwood and walk up the lawn to the tall monument shaped like a concave triangle. Telegraph inventor Samuel Morse is buried here with his brothers. Take Highwood down to Orchard Ave. and go left.

● With Crescent Dell on your left and Tulip Path to your right, watch on the right for a big tree at the avenue's edge. Next to it, George Kerr's grave shows his fireman's helmet, ax, and hose. Firefighter graves in Green-Wood often signify the deceased's vocation. The fire department is also honored with several monuments, including one from 1848 near Kerr portraying a fireman rescuing a child. Another profession well represented in the cemetery is baseball. The game's first superstar, James Creighton Jr., is buried on your right. Creighton was a fearsome pitcher and slugger who played for the Niagaras and the Excelsiors, two of the many pro clubs fielded in Brooklyn in the mid-1800s. He died at age 21 of a ruptured bladder, said to be caused by his swinging too hard at the baseball. Across the avenue, Adsit children are memorialized with lambs and an empty chair with a cloak—similar symbolism to the draped urn.

● Follow Orchard around to the left, then go left on Crescent Ave., walking beside Dell Water and then Crescent Water. Go onto Dale Ave., then right on Vernal Ave. Turn left at Union Ave., then right on Southwood Ave. Stay to the left as the road curves and becomes Locust Ave. Across from Circlet Path, beside a large tree, an urn atop a pillar is surrounded by low headstones. These are Colgate graves—as in toothpaste. Shortly after them on the left is a grave with a fireman's helmet and hose. OUR LOST COMRADE are virtually the only legible words in the inscription.

● Go right on Violet Path, then right on Circlet Path. On your right you'll pass the grave of James Merritt Ives, printer of iconic pictures of wintertime idylls. Keep walking around Circlet to Fir Path and go left, then go right on Vista Ave. After Southwood, this will take you onto Grape Ave. At its intersection with Locust, two stone posts to your left identify a Roosevelt plot. Among those buried here are Martha and Alice Roosevelt, the mother and first wife of Teddy Roosevelt. He was serving in the New York State Assembly—his first public office—when he rushed home after his wife took ill following childbirth. Upon arrival, he discovered that his mother's cold had escalated to typhoid. The women died in the same house on the same day in 1884. The Roosevelt graves are largely illegible, but you can make out THEODORE on those of Alice and Martha.

●  Across Grape Ave. from the Roosevelts, follow Hazel Path all the way to Vernal Ave. and turn right. Watch on your left for the Moorish mausoleum of industrialist Cornelius Garrison, 1853–54 mayor of San Francisco who got rich on the gold rush and Mississippi River steamboats. He later moved to New York and headed shipping and rail concerns.

●  Walk up Jonquil Path behind Garrison's mausoleum and turn right on Cypress Ave. Then go left on Dale. Turn right on Sassafras Ave. to see the enormous sword-bearing angel sitting on the Rinelli Guardino mausoleum. Then go back on Sassafras—a playful name that doesn't prepare you for the startling image coming up after you turn right on Dale: a bride reclining beneath the cross of the Merello Volta grave. Little is known about the deceased, but unconfirmed rumors say she was a Mafia bride whacked on her wedding day. Brace yourself for another creepy sculpture after you turn left from Dale onto Fir. (Before you reach it, you can detour left on Mistletoe Path and look amid the row of simple, low-lying graves to your right for Jean-Michel Basquiat, artist and protégé of Andy Warhol.) To your left on Fir is another representation of the angel of death—a cloak without a body inside. It marks the grave of Charles and Mary Schieren, who died a day apart in 1915. He was a former mayor of Brooklyn.

●  Turn left on Grape. Immediately after Lychis Path on your right, find the Wuppermann graves. There are at least five men named Frank Morgan buried in Green-Wood, but only the one born Francis Wuppermann played the title role in one of the greatest movies of all time, *The Wizard of Oz.*

●  Go right on Sassafras Ave., right on Lonicera Path, and then left on Fir. Turn right on Vine Ave., lined with all kinds of intriguing statuary. Turn left on Border Ave., another prime avenue for extravagant burial sites. They include (to your right) a long bench where a forlorn lass sits and, across from it, the temple-esque tomb of Charles Feltman, with cupola and angel on top. Feltman was a Coney Island restaurateur who came up with the idea to put a sausage in a bun for eating without silverware—and the hot dog was born.

●  Continue on Border to the Hillside Mausoleum at Cypress Ave., where you can take a break. Upholstered seats are just one luxury in this 21st-century addition to Green-

Wood. The building also features a five-story atrium, pyramid skylights, reflecting pools, Tibetan wool carpets, and recorded music. Floor-to-ceiling windows provide sweeping views.

- Exit the mausoleum on level 3, onto Dawn Path. On your right is the squat, plain grave of celebrity clergyman and liberal firebrand Henry Ward Beecher, who preached in Brooklyn Heights for nearly 40 years. He lies with his wife; his mistress, Elizabeth Tilton, is buried elsewhere in Green-Wood. Throughout the rabidly publicized scandal of their affair, Beecher refused to acknowledge he had behaved immorally, and his epitaph indicates he took that conviction to the grave. As you head down Dawn, the cut-stone grave bearing a female statue belongs to another old-time baseball star, Richard T. Godwin, the No. 1 catcher in pro ball in the 1850s. At Dawn's intersection with Hillside is the pyramid tomb of Henry Bergh, founder of the American Society for the Prevention of Cruelty to Animals. He died in 1888; just recently, a metal mural of animals was laid in front of him.

- Go right on Hillside. The churchlike mausoleum on your left at Ocean was built for John Mackay, a Scottish immigrant who made a fortune mining in Nevada during the gold rush and then augmented it with railroad and telegraph investments on the East Coast. He and his wife lived as profligately as they have been laid to rest—in a heated marble tomb adorned with bronze statues that cost him over $4 million in today's dollars. Go left on Mountain Path across from the Mackay tomb, past several dramatic Gothic monuments, and turn right at the Allen grave. Walk on the grass to showman Imre Kiralfy's stained-glass mausoleum. Look inside it to see how pretty the windows are.

*A grave near Landscape and Oak Aves.*

- Return to the Mackays, and walk on Ocean with their tomb on your left. Make the first right onto Atlantic Ave. and follow it to a loop. Halfway around, go onto Grove Ave. to your left, then right onto Central Ave. On your right where Central meets Larch Ave., behind a reclining woman with headless child, you can see the tall grave of Charles Pfizer, whose name is on a Fortune 500 company that started in Brooklyn. Stay on Central to the next avenue, where you can go right. Take that to Atlantic Ave. and go left. Watch for the Badger and Wilcox monuments on your right. Look about four rows behind them to a statue of a drummer boy. This is the grave of Clarence Mackenzie, a regiment drummer who was the first Brooklynite to give his life in the Civil War. He was 12 years old. Many Civil War veterans are buried in this area, as well as a 19th-century artist named William Beard. You shouldn't have any trouble finding his grave a little farther along on Atlantic. It's guarded by his favorite subject—the bear. He often painted them dancing.

- Follow Atlantic Ave. onto Meadow Ave. and then back onto Atlantic. Turn left on Hydrangea Path and watch immediately for the Griffith grave. On the side facing away from Hydrangea, husband Charles had his last memory of JANE MY WIFE sculpted in marble, saying goodbye to him outside their Greenwich Village townhouse. She died while he was at work. Continue on Hydrangea to Fern Ave. and go left. On your left at Greenbough Ave., an elaborate altar with weeping angels memorializes Charlotte Canda. The only child of a Napoleonic officer who had immigrated to New York, Charlotte was killed when she was thrown from a carriage after the horses pulling it were startled by a storm. She was on her way home from her 17th birthday party.

- Go right on Greenbough. A gray obelisk on a hill to your right, behind two crosses, marks the grave of Henry Raymond, founder of *The New York Times.* He also cofounded the Republican Party, which today considers *The Times* an enemy combatant.

- Go left at Sycamore Ave., where Rex the dog sits, appropriately, beside a tree. Return to Greenbough and go to the left around the loop, turning right onto Cypress Path on the other side. A small, worn grave on your left belongs to William Merritt Chase, the American impressionist who painted many Brooklyn scenes. At Myrtle Path, ascend to the Pierreponts' hill and the Gothic Revival brownstone structure (by Richard Upjohn) that's been described as an "open-air church." Henry Pierrepont was behind the creation of Green-Wood.

- Go left back onto Myrtle. Turn right on the path that takes you across Central Ave. and onto Sycamore, and turn left. Turn right on Rue Path, then go left onto Bay Grove. Follow that path around to the oval dominated by the statue of DeWitt Clinton, mayor of New York City, governor of New York State, U.S. senator, and runner-up to James Madison in the 1812 presidential election. Clinton was buried in the state capital of Albany upon his death in 1828, and his 1853 reinterment at Green-Wood was a masterstroke of publicity for the fledgling cemetery. Across the path from Clinton's grave, the statue of a child (called Little Frankie) was crafted by Daniel Chester French, who sculpted Lincoln for the Lincoln Memorial. Clinton himself looks down on the grave of printmaker Nathaniel Currier, buried with his two wives and infant children.

- Walk up Bayside Path behind Clinton's grave. Turn right and, shortly after, left on Highland Ave. Turn left at Fern Ave., where you have a view of the Williamsburgh Savings Bank clocktower to your left. Go up the second staircase on your right to the Pilot's Monument, erected at the grave of ship pilot Thomas Freeborn, who perished when his vessel was battered by a storm in New York Harbor. The incident is depicted on the sarcophagus, and above it a mast with its top cut off alludes to Freeborn's premature death. Fittingly, this spot offers a superb view across the harbor.

- From Fern Ave., turn right on Mulberry Ave. and then left on Hemlock Ave. On your left at the intersection with Battle Ave., the bust on a pedestal marks the grave of Elias Howe Jr., inventor of the sewing machine. Behind the bust is the grave of Fannie, a dog, inscribed with a verse countering those who might question the fuss over "only a dog." Proceed on Hemlock across Garland Ave. To your left, behind the Seamans tomb, sits the modest grave of Juan Trippe, founder of Pan Am Airways, who was portrayed by Alec Baldwin in the 2004 movie *The Aviator.* Farther along on your left, the decorous resting place of John Torrio belies his conduct in life. Born in Italy, he ran Chicago's prostitution and bootlegging rackets before Al Capone.

- Turn left on Border Ave. and follow it around to Garland Ave. Turn left and, opposite the grave of Charles H. Ebbets, owner of the Brooklyn Dodgers, go right on Battle Path. A bronze statue of Minerva, the Roman goddess of battle, stands at the altar of liberty, in a tribute to the Battle of Brooklyn, which was fought on this hill. It was positioned so Liberty is waving to Liberty—turn around when you're in front of Minerva and look across the harbor to understand.

- Go left on Liberty Path and look for the in-ground gravestone of composer/conductor Leonard Bernstein, who's buried with his wife and sister. Visitors usually leave stones on the grave—a way of paying respects to the dead in Judaism. Bernstein is one of the few Jews in Green-Wood.

- Go back to Battle Path and turn left. The Soldiers' Monument is a proud achievement of Green-Wood and one of the earliest Civil War memorials, erected in 1869. It honors the 148,000 New Yorkers who fought for the Union with statues of a cavalryman (with sword), engineer (ax), infantryman (gun), and artilleryman. They're on a hill that's the highest natural point in Brooklyn.

- At Battle Ave., across from Battle Hill, a dead man tells a tale: the temperance diatribe on R.H. McDonald's grave boasts that he abstained from liquor and tobacco for the last 40 years of his life. But he lived to 83, so who knows what carousing he did when he was young. Go right on Battle.

- On Battle Ave. near Bayview Ave., a Sphinx guards a pyramid whose doorway is flanked by Jesus and Mary. Originally, a bronze image of the Egyptian sun god Ra was affixed behind the Sphinx, where there's now just a splotch. This tomb was the brainchild of Albert Parsons, a music teacher and fan of Egyptiana. A different kind of temple forms the tomb of John Anderson, farther along Battle to your left. He chose a Greek design to represent his democratic ideals. Anderson, who made his money in tobacco, helped finance Garibaldi's crusade in Italy and other causes. If you walk on the grass behind Anderson, you'd come to Frederick A.O. Schwarz, namesake of the 5th Ave. toy emporium. In this part of Battle Ave., you'll also see the elaborate plots of the Burr and Spencer families.

- On your right, where both Bayside and Bayview Aves. meet Battle Ave., stands a memorial to those lost in the Brooklyn Theater fire of 1876. The fire broke out backstage just as the play was ending and quickly spread throughout the theater, claiming 278 lives. Kate Claxton, who starred in the play (and survived the fire), is buried in Green-Wood not far from the Roosevelts. Already a popular stage actress, she become a household name after the fire.

- On your left at Arbor Ave., note the serene angels sculpted in bronze on the Stewart mausoleum as well as the cherub faces along the top. The tomb was designed by architect Stanford White and sculptor Augustus Saint-Gaudens, who collaborated on several renowned monuments nationwide. The Stewarts were the parents of Isabella Stewart Gardner, patron of the arts whose private collection became Boston's premier art museum.

- Battle Ave. takes you back to the main gate, one block from the R train at 25th St. and 4th Ave.

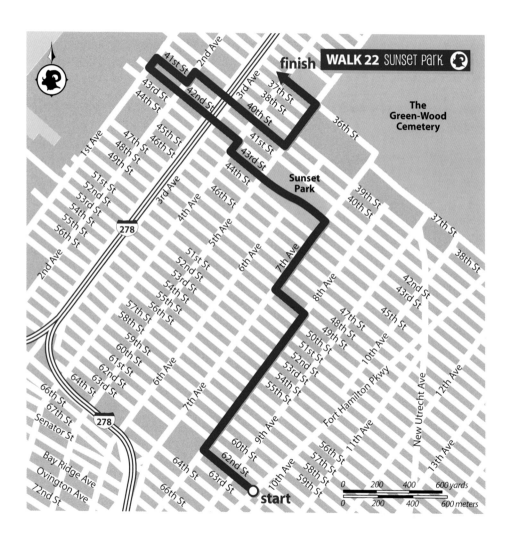

WALK 22 SUNSET PARK

finish

The Green-Wood Cemetery

Sunset Park

start

# 22 SUNSET PARK: MELTING POT ON THE WATERFRONT

**BOUNDARIES: Fort Hamilton Pkwy., 8th Ave., 36th St., 1st Ave.**
**DISTANCE: Approx. 3 miles**
**SUBWAY: N to Fort Hamilton Pkwy.**

On one Saturday every June, the flags of over 50 nations are proudly hoisted, waved, and applauded during Sunset Park's Parade of Flags, a celebration unique to this polyglot neighborhood. Sunset Park has been an ethnic enclave for nearly two centuries, with populations shifting and overlapping through different waves of immigration. Now flavored by Chinese, Latino, Turkish, and Southeast Asian residents, it still bears influences from the Scandinavians, Italians, Irish, and Poles who lived here en masse in past generations. Sunset Park also has been shaped by economic trends. The southern terminus of Brooklyn's industrial waterfront, it bustled with commercial activity in the first half of the 20th century. After a period of decline, the area near the water has been reborn as a manufacturing center. New companies are filling facilities such as the Cass Gilbert–designed Brooklyn Army Terminal, which was—during its military service from 1919 to 1970—the point of departure for nearly every American who served in Europe during World War II. Most homes in Sunset Park were built by the early 20th century, and several streets are lined with uniform rows of houses with bow or bay windows and embellished cornices.

● Turn left onto Fort Hamilton Pkwy. upon leaving the subway station, then turn right on 62nd St. Most signage here is in Chinese, but Norwegian flags are flying near #850, whose door is marked MEMBERS ONLY. This is home base for Sporting Club Gjøa, a soccer club founded around 1912. There used to be many more of them in this neighborhood, which has been nicknamed Little Norway and Finntown over the years. The Norwegian Folk Dance Society of New York practices at the club. If you look over your left shoulder as you near 8th Ave., you'll see its name painted on the side of the building. A few blocks to the south and west from here—away from where we're headed—is a city park named for Leif Ericson that contains a replica of a Viking rune dedicated by Norway's Crown Prince Olav when he visited in 1939.

● Turn right on 8th Ave. and proceed into the heart of Brooklyn's Chinatown. But wait, there's a mosque here on the right between 60th and 59th Sts.! And in another instance of Sunset Park's multicultural heritage, it's in a building that used to be an Irish dance club. Faith Camii, which is also the headquarters of the United American Muslim Association of New York, welcomes visitors. Imported Turkish tile adorns walls and the fountain where worshippers wash before prayers.

- The fish and seafood markets of Chinatown, while impressive in selection and price, can be unsettling for some palates—what with tanks of eels and whole squid among the merchandise. At Sea Town, on your left at 58th St., the vats of live animals for cooking include frogs and turtles. Chinese don't come to 8th Ave.—or, as they call it, Bat Dai Do (Big 8th St.)—just for food. Everything from insurance to toys and electronics are sold here. There's also a Malaysian and Vietnamese presence on the avenue.

- Turn left on 49th St., a street not dissimilar from its neighbors but which also has the more evocative name Sunset Terr. If it's flower season, look for a pretty garden between #753 and #747.

- Turn right at 7th Ave., passing two 90-year-old churches that now serve Spanish-speaking parishioners. Enormous St. Agatha's also has Chinese services. On your left near 47th St. is a botanica, a type of store found in Hispanic neighborhoods that stocks folk-religion paraphernalia like herbs, perfumes, and masks.

- At 44th St., the park that gave this neighborhood its name is on your left, opposite P.S. 169, which has occupied this imposing building for nearly 100 years. Enter Sunset Park up the steps between 43rd and 42nd Sts. If the recreation center is open, go inside to see murals by local schoolchildren as well as the Art Deco ticket booth and locker-room signs. The building and pool were Works Progress Administration projects, opened in the summer of 1936.

- From the rec center, go to your left (or to your right if you didn't go inside and are facing the building). Follow the path toward the flagpole, which was erected after the park's carousel was removed. It is remembered with imprints of carousel horses in the pavement. Wander around the park as much as you'd like. The bench-lined alley of trees is especially inviting when leaves are on the trees. Sitting as it is on a 200-foot-high hill, the park offers sweeping views of the harbor, including the Manhattan skyline, Statue of Liberty, and New Jersey. Walk down the path closest to 44th St. to where it intersects with the second-lowest path. This may be the only place where you can see the tallest buildings of Manhattan, Queens, and Brooklyn all at once. They are, from left, the Empire State, Citibank (shiny and modern), and the Williamsburgh Savings Bank clocktower.

- Leave the park at 43rd St. via the grand staircase with masonry urns at top and bottom. You can go left on 5th Ave. for a block and a half to International Restaurant for some satisfying home cooking, Dominican-style. Return to 43rd and walk down Nicholas J. Sciarra Pl., named in honor of a 41-year-old Community Board member who choked to death on a sandwich during a board meeting in 1993. The Community Board has its offices in the Classical Revival former courthouse on your right at 4th Ave. It was designed in 1931 by an architect who had a hand in Grand Central Terminal, and it should also be viewed from 42nd St. Diagonally across from it at 43rd St. is perhaps the saddest orphan in New York City architecture. This Romanesque "castle" is listed on the National Register of Historic Places as the 68th Police Precinct Station House and Stable (though it was built in 1892 for the 18th Precinct). The Sunset Park School of Music was supposed to become its first tenant in over 20 years but never moved in. Try to appreciate it despite the graffiti and scaffolding.

- Go to the right on 4th Ave. until you are beneath St. Michael's, the church that was visible from the park. This 1905 church is often likened to Paris's Sacré-Coeur and extends nearly to 3rd Ave.

- Go left on 42nd St. and cross 3rd Ave., a thoroughfare that was virtually doomed by the construction of the Gowanus Expressway in the early 1960s. This avenue had been the social and commercial heart of Sunset

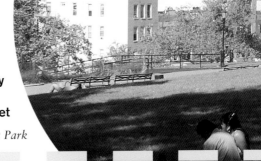

*View from Sunset Park*

Park before Robert Moses's highway rendered it undesirable to most everyone except drug dealers and porn merchants—and cost 1,000 people their homes. It has improved somewhat since then, with respectable if unaesthetic businesses setting up shop, but the rupture between industrial and residential districts was permanent.

- Proceed to 2nd Ave. From here to the water and for about 8 blocks to your left and roughly 14 to your right, this was all Bush Terminal, a complex that drove Sunset Park's economy for decades. Twenty-five shipping lines used the 18 piers and 22-block spread of warehouses of Bush Terminal, which had been considered a boondoggle when oil scion Irving T. Bush conceived it in 1890. Some of its buildings, such as those you see in both directions on 2nd, still possess an elegance, though they're slightly shabby. Continue to 1st Ave. The warehouse on the left at #4201, built in 1890, resembles a medieval fortress. You can't see its Gothic tower from 42nd, so look back after turning right on 1st. Now that the Bush Terminal space has been revived for industry, politicians and residents have turned their attention to the waterfront's recreation potential.

- Turn right on 1st Ave. Those tracks are remnants of the dedicated railroad that served the Bush Terminal, which also had its own power plant, police force, and fire department. Turn right on 41st St. and keep following the old tracks to the left on 2nd Ave. Then turn right on 40th St. As you may observe, products from ice cream to shoes to paint are now being manufactured in Sunset Park. When you reach 3rd Ave., on your left is one of the only retailers that survived the expressway construction. Frankel's has been in business since 1890, when it opened as a sort of general store for dock workers.

- Continuing up 40th St., you'll pass another distinguished-looking school on 4th Ave. to your right. This junior high has had standardized-testing and discipline problems, but all looks fine on the outside, with its ornamented triangular parapets. Across 4th, both sides of 40th have rows of refined houses with columned entryways.

- Turn left on 5th Ave., *la calle principal* for the Latino population of Sunset Park. Puerto Ricans were the first Latinos to arrive in the area, starting in the 1950s, but nowadays more residents come from Mexico, Ecuador, the Dominican Republic, and

Central America. There are also Chinese businesses on this street—and some cultural hybrids, like the restaurants serving "comida China."

● The walk ends at a bus depot, not for a ride but to see a tribute: to TV legend Jackie Gleason, who made Brooklyn and bus drivers proud with his portrayal of blustery Brooklyn busman Ralph Kramden on *The Honeymooners.* The depot was renamed for the Brooklyn native a year after he died, and the *Honeymooners* logo appears in both the blue-and-white sign and the metal plaque below it on the building near 36th St.

● Turn left on 36th St. to reach the D, N, or R train at 4th Ave.

## POINTS OF INTEREST

**Faith Camii mosque** 5911 8th Ave., Brooklyn, NY 11220, 718-438-6919
**Sunset Park** 5th to 7th Aves. between 41st and 44th Sts., Brooklyn, NY 11220
**International Restaurant** 4408 5th Ave., Brooklyn, NY 11220, 718-438-2009
**Frankel's** 3924 3rd Ave., Brooklyn, NY 11232, 718-768-9788

## route summary

1. From the Fort Hamilton Pkwy. station, turn right on 62nd St.
2. Turn right on 8th Ave.
3. Turn left on 49th St.
4. Turn right on 7th Ave.
5. Enter Sunset Park between 43rd and 42nd Sts. Exit on 5th Ave.
6. Walk west on 43rd.
7. Turn right on 4th Ave.
8. Go left on 42nd.
9. Turn right on 1st Ave., right on 41st St., left on 2nd Ave., and right on 40th St.
10. Go left on 5th Ave.
11. Go left on 36th St. to the subway at 4th Ave.

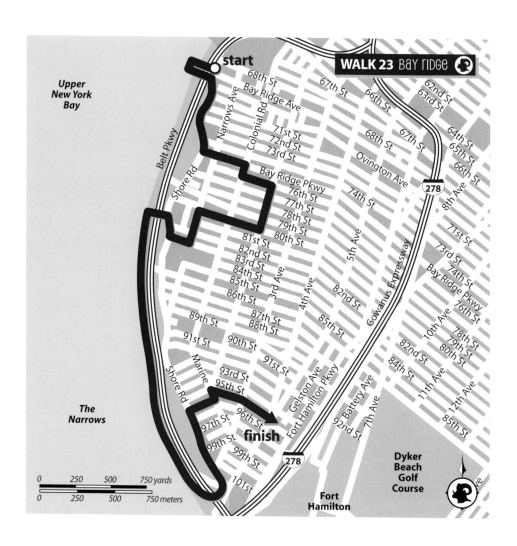

start

**WALK 23** Bay Ridge

Upper
New York
Bay

68th St
67th St
62nd St
63rd St
Bay Ridge Ave
66th St
Narrows Ave
Colonial Rd
71st St
68th St
67th St
64th St
72nd St
Ovington Ave
65th St
73rd St
66th St
Belt Pkwy
Shore Rd
Bay Ridge Pkwy
74th St
278
8th Ave
76th St
77th St
71st St
78th St
5th Ave
73rd St
79th St
74th St
80th St
Bay Ridge Pkwy
81st St
76th St
82nd St
3rd Ave
4th Ave
Gowanus Expressway
10th Ave
78th St
83rd St
82nd St
79th St
84th St
80th St
85th St
85th St
86th St
11th Ave
87th St
89th St
88th St
12th Ave
91st St
90th St
82nd St
85th St
Shore Rd
91st St
93rd St
84th St
Marine
95th St
Gelston Ave
Battery Ave
The
Narrows
96th St
Fort Hamilton Pkwy
92nd St
7th Ave
Dyker
Beach
Golf
Course
**finish**
97th St
99th St
99th St
278
101st
Fort
Hamilton

0    250    500    750 yards
0    250    500    750 meters

178

# 23 Bay Ridge: Mansions in the Shadow of a Great Bridge

**BOUNDARIES:** Bay Ridge Ave., shore path, 4th Ave.
**DISTANCE:** Approx. 3½ miles
**SUBWAY:** R to Bay Ridge Ave., transfer to B1 bus to Bay Ridge

Unlike many Brooklyn neighborhoods with "Hill" in their name, Bay Ridge actually sits on elevated ground—a bluff overlooking Upper New York Bay. It was the proximity to and views of the water that attracted Manhattan's elite in the late 1800s, when Bay Ridge developed as a summer resort. The extension of the subway system in 1915 opened the neighborhood to the middle class, and it became more urbanized. Few mansions remain from the early years, though there are many large freestanding modern houses. Ethnically, Bay Ridge has long been identified with Italian-Americans (who supplanted Scandinavians as the predominant group) and more recently has gained Russian and Middle Eastern populations. Throughout the years it has remained one of the best places in Brooklyn to enjoy the water. This walk stays close to the shore and thus bypasses the lively commercial district farther inland that's centered around 86th St. and 5th Ave., where you'd find plenty of mom-and-pop businesses, Italian restaurants, and Irish pubs.

● Bay Ridge Ave. is one of those formal street names (like Manhattan's Avenue of the Americas) generally forsaken by locals in favor of the numerical designation—in this case, 69th St. Ride the bus to Shore Rd., then walk straight ahead onto the 600-foot-long pier. You're bound to see fishermen, kids running around, and maybe even some people using the picnic tables for what they were intended for. The view of the Verrazano-Narrows Bridge is awesome, but the unique vantage point here is of the Hudson River—New Jersey to the west, Manhattan to its east—as it empties into Upper New York Bay. Miss Liberty's in the picture too. Gazing full-on at Manhattan's southern tip, you can just imagine the spectacular view of the Twin Towers this pier used to offer, which is why Brooklyn's 9/11 memorial is here. It's shaped like a fire-fighter's trumpet—used in the 18th century, as sirens are today, to warn of a fire. Also in honor of 9/11, the pier was formally named American Veterans Memorial Pier.

- Go back to Shore Rd. and turn right, walking alongside Shore Road Park. This northern end of the 58-acre park encompasses Narrows Botanical Garden, a decade-old volunteer project. Enter at 71st St., just past the lily pond, and walk through a linden-tree alley, then go to your right and follow the path around the lawn, enjoying the flowers and redwood trees. You can take a path north of the lawn to the native-plant section, which is an officially designated turtle sanctuary. Heading south from the lawn, walk on the path nearer the water and you'll find a butterfly garden on your right.

- Stay on the path and it will take you back to Shore Rd. at 72nd St. Go to your right on Shore. A little farther along, look across the ball fields at the Verrazano-Narrows Bridge. You'll see more of it—getting closer and closer—as the walk progresses, but this view of one tower above the trees in the park is a worthwhile photo op.

- Proceed on Shore Rd. to Bay Ridge Pkwy. (75th St.) and turn left. You've entered the approximately eight-by-three-block area where Bay Ridge's grandest homes are concentrated.

- Turn right on Colonial Rd., then go left on 76th St. and ascend the staircase. The "ridge" at this point was too steep for vehicles, so the steps were installed to accommodate pedestrians. Two original mansions are at the top of the stairs. On the left, #131, with its circular columned porch, dates to 1865. The house opposite it at #122 with a hexagonal tower was built in 1900 (for the founder of Blue Cross).

- Turn right on Ridge Blvd. and proceed to 80th St. Union Church, whose impressive stained glass is visible from outside, was founded when a Dutch Reformed church on the site merged with a Presbyterian church located a block away. The combined congregation built this church in 1924, but the front of the sanctuary comprises the original Reformed structure of 1896.

- Turn right on 80th and go left at Narrows Ave. Around here, homes are adorned with such special features as etched glass panes, lion sentinels, and multitiered birdbaths. One fanciful house and its expansive lawn occupy the entire west side of the block from 82nd to 83rd Sts. Nicknamed the Gingerbread House, the Howard E. and Jessie Jones House was built in 1916 and is one of New York's few specimens of the Arts and Crafts movement of that era. With a fake thatched roof, it resembles a cottage out of a fairy tale.

- Turn right on 83rd and right again on Shore Rd. Note the trilevel fountain on the grounds at 82nd, as well as the white-lattice balcony on the house, which is enclosed by a marble fence. Another super-sumptuous abode is at 80th, and just past it the property at #7925 features a mini-windmill.

- Across Shore Rd., the flagstaff with yardarm honors the Spanish-American War victory and goes by the moniker Old Glory Lookout. Walk downhill via either path next to it, then cross over the Belt Pkwy. to the water's edge.

- This paved path that hugs the shoreline is one of NYC's best places for biking, Rollerblading, or just bench-sitting with a view. And, of course, for walking. Head south until you are almost beneath the Verrazano-Narrows Bridge. John Travolta wooed his leading lady here in a scene in *Saturday Night Fever,* whose hero lived (and boogied) in Bay Ridge.

- Take the last path to your left before the bridge and walk uphill; it leads onto a sidewalk that puts you back on Shore Rd. Cross Shore and go to the left to check out Fontbonne Hall Academy at 99th St. This onetime villa—the only 19th-century home still standing on Shore Rd.—was built as a summer estate and later purchased by corpulent railroad tycoon Diamond Jim Brady for his showgirl paramour Lillian Russell.

- Turn right on 95th St. A few doors in on your left, the pale yellow house with green shutters and a lovely porch

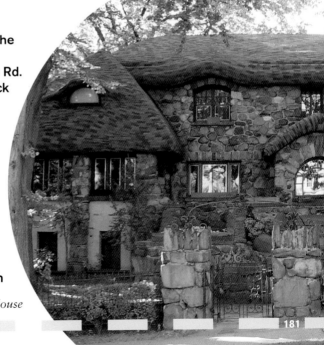

*The Gingerbread House*

is the oldest house in Bay Ridge, sitting here since it was surrounded by farmland in 1849.

● Continue on 95th, zigzagging to the left and right at Marine Ave. to stay on 95th. Bay Ridge has always been a place for Irish pubs, so have a drink or meal at the one to your right on 3rd Ave., Ballybunion. Or, for a quick bite on 3rd Ave., go to Bake Ridge Bagels to the left off 95th. Walk one block more on 95th to 4th Ave. for the R train.

## POINTS OF INTEREST

**American Veterans Memorial Pier** 69th St. at Shore Rd., Brooklyn, NY 11209

**Narrows Botanical Garden** Shore Rd. between Bay Ridge Ave. and 72nd St., Brooklyn, NY 11209

**Ballybunion** 9510 3rd Ave., Brooklyn, NY 11209, 718-833-2801

**Bake Ridge Bagels** 9417 3rd Ave., Brooklyn, NY 11209, 718-680-6353

## ROUTE SUMMARY

1. Begin at Shore Rd. and 69th St. and walk onto the pier.
2. Return to Shore Rd. and turn right.
3. Go into Narrows Botanical Garden on your right at 71st St.
4. Exit the garden at 72nd St. and continue south on Shore Rd.
5. Turn left on Bay Ridge Pkwy.
6. Turn right on Colonial Rd., then left on 76th St.
7. Turn right on Ridge Blvd.
8. Turn right on 80th St., then left at Narrows Ave.
9. Turn right on 83rd St. and right again on Shore Rd.
10. From Old Glory Lookout, use the walkway to get to the waterside path and go left.
11. Take the path on the left just before the bridge to return to Shore Rd. and turn left.
12. Turn right on 95th St. and proceed to the subway at 4th Ave.

*The Verrazano-Narrows Bridge from 4th Ave.*

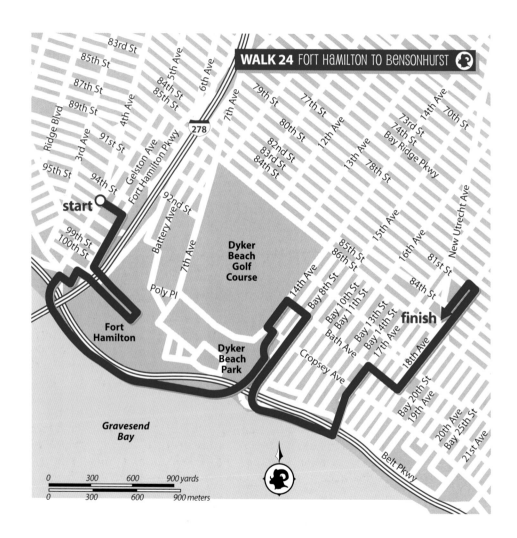

83rd St
85th St
87th St
89th St

5th Ave
6th Ave

84th St
85th St

7th Ave

79th St
80th St
82nd St
83rd St
84th St

77th St
12th Ave

73rd St
74th St
14th Ave
70th St
Bay Ridge Pkwy

Ridge Blvd

4th Ave
3rd Ave
91st St

95th St
94th St

Gelston Ave
Fort Hamilton Pkwy

278

13th Ave
78th St

New Utrecht Ave

**start**

92nd St

Battery Ave

99th St
100th St

7th Ave

Poly Pl

**Dyker
Beach
Golf
Course**

15th Ave
16th Ave
81st St

**Fort
Hamilton**

14th Ave

85th St
86th St

Bay 8th St
Bay 10th St
Bay 11th St

84th St

**finish**

**Dyker
Beach
Park**

Bath Ave

Bay 13th St
Bay 14th St
17th Ave

18th Ave

Cropsey Ave

*Gravesend
Bay*

Bay 20th St
19th Ave

20th Ave
Bay 25th St
21st Ave

Belt Pkwy

| 0 | 300 | 600 | 900 yards |
| 0 | 300 | 600 | 900 meters |

# 24 FOrT HamILTON TO BeNSONHUrST: Bay WaTCH, ITaLIan-STYLe

**BOUNDARIES: 4th Ave., shore path, 18th Ave., 81st St.**
**DISTANCE: Approx. 5 miles**
**SUBWAY: R to 95th St.**

New Utrecht was one of the five original towns established by the Dutch in the 17th century in what would eventually become the city, then borough, of Brooklyn. This walk includes present-day neighborhoods within the area once under the jurisdiction of New Utrecht. The route hugs the shoreline as you go from neighborhood to neighborhood via the off-street biking/walking path along Lower New York Bay (aka Gravesend Bay). While this is intended mostly as a scenic walk, it's bookended by two places of historical significance: Fort Hamilton and what remains of New Utrecht. Even if you've never heard of the communities this walk travels through—Dyker Heights, Bath Beach—you know their inhabitants: those traditional working-class Italian-Americans portrayed (and stereotyped) in countless movies and TV shows. *Andiamo!*

- From the subway, walk on 4th Ave. toward the Verrazano-Narrows Bridge. You're in the neighborhood of Fort Hamilton, the part of Bay Ridge closest to the military post of Fort Hamilton. This area used to be nicknamed Irishtown, as Irish people started settling here in the 1820s. Bay Ridge still has its own St. Patrick's Day parade. Not surprisingly, it starts at St. Patrick's Church, which has stood at the corner of 4th Ave. and 95th St. since 1925. Turn left on 95th at the church.

- Turn right on Fort Hamilton Pkwy. In *Saturday Night Fever,* John Travolta and pals hung out in this park beneath the bridge. This area also gets screen time every November when the New York City Marathon is televised and the runners pour into Brooklyn via those bridge access lanes you can see from Fort Hamilton Pkwy.

- You wouldn't expect to find Confederate history in Brooklyn, but it's here on your right at 99th St. St. John's Church, which looks like a house, is where Episcopalians stationed at Fort Hamilton have worshipped. That includes Confederate generals Robert

E. Lee, who served the church as a vestryman in the early 1840s, and Stonewall Jackson, who was baptized here after graduating from West Point and fighting in the Mexican-American War. All that actually happened in the original St. John's, which was founded in 1834; this structure was built on the same site in 1890.

- At 101st St., enter Fort Hamilton—the second-oldest (after West Point) continuously garrisoned fort in the United States, used primarily at present for recruitment and new-enlistee processing. A battery on this site was deployed strategically in the American Revolution and War of 1812, and construction on the current fort began in 1825. Robert E. Lee was the garrison's chief engineer from 1841 to 1846.

- After going through security, proceed to Sterling Dr. and turn right. The sextet of large houses you see across the lawn is known as Colonel's Row because guess who got to live there. Artillery from various countries and eras lines the walkway on your left. Turn left at Sheridan Loop and go inside the Fort Hamilton Community Club on your right. Originally the main fort, this building was converted to an officers' club in 1938 and today is a membership club for federal employees. The corridors and niches that remain from the old fort structure make for interesting exploring, complete with historical maps, photos, and military and household objects. The Harbor Defense Museum is the next stop, farther along Sheridan Loop on your left. Admission is free, and its collection spans two centuries of New York military history. Go left when you leave the museum, then right at the cannonball pyramid. When you reach the clubhouse pool, take the uphill path across from it, on your left. Walk past the cannon and basketball courts to the farther end of the bluff. Enjoy a respite on a bench overlooking a vast expanse of water. You can see Coney Island's high-rises and Parachute Jump to your left and Staten Island beaches to your right. Retrace your route in reverse to exit Fort Hamilton.

- When you leave the fort, go straight ahead on 101st and enter John Paul Jones Park on your left at 4th Ave. Ahead, about 50 cannonballs are stacked around a Rodman gun. This cannon was the largest gun used in the Civil War (after being tested at Fort Hamilton), and very few still exist. On the other side of the lawn, a low-lying monument recognizes the efforts of one John LaCorte to promote the achievements of Italian-Americans; thanks to Signor LaCorte, the bridge above you is named not only for the water it traverses (the Narrows strait links Upper and Lower New York Bay), but also for the Italian who was the first European explorer to sail into New York Harbor. About 8,000 residents of Bay Ridge/Fort Hamilton—including a lot of Italian-Americans—were displaced when the bridge was erected in 1964. It was the world's longest (4,260 feet) suspension bridge at the time and is still the longest in the United States.

● From the park, cross 4th Ave. and go to your left. Cross Shore Rd. and take the path downhill (not into Shore Road Park), which will lead onto the sidewalk along the Belt Pkwy. E. At the bottom of the hill, cross over to the shore path and go left. Walk under the bridge, noting the reef that anchors it on this side. An island fort named Lafayette, opened in 1818, was demolished to make room for those bridge supports. The abandoned (and polluted) jetty marked U.S. ARMY that you pass just after the bridge was Denyse Wharf, a landing point for the Brits in the Battle of Brooklyn. It was later part of Fort Hamilton and then a ferry terminal whose services were no longer needed once the bridge opened. You'll find more information about Denyse Wharf on signs placed by the New York Aquarium. Watch on your right for these IT HAPPENED HERE markers, which also describe Brooklyn's geological origins and a couple of lesser-known islands in New York Bay.

● When you come to stairs on your left, take them to cross over the highway, and then cross one of its on-ramps to Bay 8th St. and turn right. Walk through Dyker Beach Park, the western extension of Dyker Heights—a residential neighborhood with few commercial establishments other than a bakery here, a pizzeria there. But it does have the second-largest city park in Brooklyn, built on top of a beach. Come out of the park on Cropsey Ave. and turn left.

*In John Paul Jones Park*

## CHRISTMASTIME IN DYKER HEIGHTS

Planning starts in July. Professionals are hired. And the results are bodacious enough to have been the subject of a PBS documentary. It's the holiday illuminations and decorations of Dyker Heights. There are nativity scenes, merry-go-rounds, enormous inflatable characters, mannequins that dance and ice skate, and piped-in music too. The homeowners of Dyker Heights are not shy about their Christmas spirit. Some of them reportedly light up as many as 10,000 bulbs on their property. Stoops, roofs, windowsills, lawns, and trees are all involved. You may see Tweety Bird and Scooby-Doo across a driveway from the Three Wise Men, or a giant snow globe tethered to a statue of Jesus that's strung with lights. These roads that are quiet 11 months of the year can get jammed with cars in December, as visitors come to see the neighborhood's limited-run, no-admission tourist attraction. To enjoy the festivities on foot, take the R train to 86th St. and transfer to the B64 bus (going toward Coney Island). Get out anywhere between 10th and 13th Aves.—within those bounds, from 86th to 80th, is the crux of the action. *Buon Natale*!

- Turn right on 14th Ave. Dyker Beach Park's public golf course is on your left; the homes on your right actually carry a Bath Beach address (except for the park, Dyker Heights is "inland"). Bath Beach was a fashionable seaside resort in the late 19th century, named after the British spa town Bath for cachet and too refined to have bars and dance halls. That's what the people wanted, though, and competition from Coney Island put Bath Beach out of business. It became residential.

- Turn right on Bath Ave., then right on Bay 8th St. Some of the big houses around here are former summer estates from the early days of Bath Beach, others are modern mansions.

- Continue on Bay 8th back toward the water, traversing the Belt Pkwy. W. on-ramp en route. Resume walking south on the shore path.

- Cross the next pedestrian bridge—it's blue—from the shore path. This will put you in Bath Beach Park, beside Bay 16th St. Follow the Joseph L. Pezzuto Walkway (you can read about its namesake's civic contributions) to 17th Ct. and proceed straight up 17th Ave.

- Turn right on Bath Ave., then turn left on 18th Ave. Sticklers will tell you you're still in Bath Beach, but to many others this is already Bensonhurst—probably the most Italian neighborhood of New York City. They even got this main drag subtitled Cristoforo Colombo Blvd., as you can see on the street signs. Italian immigrants began moving here after World War II and at one point constituted 80 percent of the population. More recently, Chinese and Russians have arrived. The unequivocal Bensonhurst boundary is 86th St. Stop in at West End Bakery on your right for a cannoli or torrone or biscotti or gelato or just about any other Italian treat you desire.

- At 85th St., look at the elevated train tracks curving from New Utrecht Ave to 86th St. One of filmdom's most famous car chases took place on these streets, the one in *The French Connection* where Gene Hackman pursues a drug dealer who's riding a train above him. A few years later, another soon-to-be iconic scene was filmed on 86th— John Travolta's opening strut of *Saturday Night Fever*. TV fans know Bensonhurst as the home of *The Honeymooners'* Ralph Kramden and the *Welcome Back, Kotter* gang.

  Back to the real world: Dutch settlers founded the New Utrecht Reformed Church, on your right on 18th Ave. between 83rd and 84th Sts., in 1677. The church has been on this site since 1699 and in this building since 1828. Its flagpole was erected in 1783 to celebrate victory in the American Revolution, thus earning the status of "liberty pole." Be sure to take a few steps off 18th to see the lovely 1892 parish house on 84th.

- Continue north on 18th, passing Garibaldi Playground on your right. Look for a monument—puzzlingly resembling a gravestone—to the Italian freedom fighter at the corner with 82nd St. Then move on to Milestone Park, another historic locale where neighborhood folks gather for multicultural gaming.

- Go back on 18th to New Utrecht Ave. for the D train. If you would like to see more of the Italian shops and social clubs, proceed on 18th through the 70s. The B8 bus will take you back to the subway.

## POINTS OF INTEREST

**Fort Hamilton's Harbor Defense Museum** 230 Sheridan Loop, Brooklyn, NY 11252, 718-630-4349

**John Paul Jones Park** 4th Ave. and 101st St., Brooklyn, NY 11209

**Dyker Beach Park** Bay 8th St. and Cropsey Ave., Brooklyn, NY 11228

**Bath Beach Park** 17th Ave. and 17th Ct., Brooklyn, NY 11214

**West End Bakery** 8517 18th Ave., Brooklyn, NY 11214, 718-259-0777

**Garibaldi Playground** 18th Ave. between 82nd and 83rd Sts., Brooklyn, NY 11214

**Milestone Park** 18th Ave. between 81st and 82nd Sts., Brooklyn, NY 11214

## ROUTE SUMMARY

1. Walk on 4th Ave. toward the Verrazano-Narrows Bridge and turn left on 95th St.
2. Turn right on Fort Hamilton Pkwy.
3. Visit Fort Hamilton at 101st St.
4. Return to 101st and leave the fort. Go straight ahead and into John Paul Jones Park.
5. Cross 4th Ave. and go left, then cross Shore Rd.
6. Walk downhill to the shore path and go left.
7. Use the pedestrian bridge to Bay 8th St.
8. Walk through Dyker Beach Park to Cropsey Ave. and go left.
9. Turn right on 14th Ave.
10. Turn right on Bath Ave. and right on Bay 8th St. to return to the shore path southbound.
11. Use the next pedestrian bridge over the highway.
12. Walk through Bath Beach Park to 17th Ave.
13. Turn right on Bath Ave., then left on 18th Ave.
14. Walk to 82nd St., then return to 18th and New Utrecht Aves. for the subway.

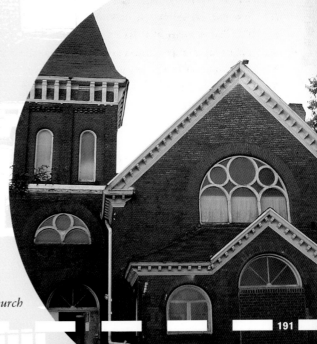

*Parish house of New Utrecht Reformed Church*

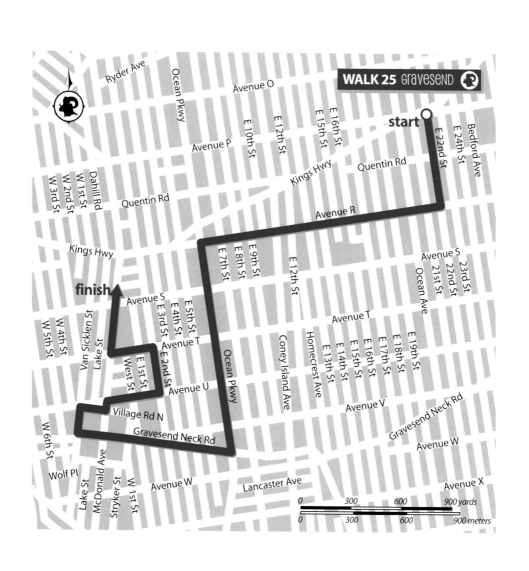

# 25 Gravesend: It Takes a Woman...

**BOUNDARIES: Kings Hwy., E. 22nd St., Gravesend Neck Rd., Van Sicklen St.**
**DISTANCE: Approx. 3¼ miles**
**SUBWAY: B or Q to Kings Hwy., transfer to the B82 bus**

One hundred and forty-four years before the United States adopted its Constitution, a town was founded on the ideals of religious, social, and political freedom and equal rights for all. It was the first of the six original settlements of Brooklyn and the only non-Dutch one among them. Most extraordinary of all, its founder was a woman: Lady Deborah Moody, a baron's widow who had left Massachusetts, her first home in the New World, because it was too restrictive—one might say puritanical—concerning personal liberties. Gravesend, the town she established in 1643 and received a land patent for in 1645, started as 28 lots on 17 acres but eventually grew to encompass the entire southern sector of present-day Brooklyn (including Coney Island). This walk explores Lady Moody's stomping grounds as well as some Dutch colonial heritage, including 4 of the 14 Dutch farmhouses still standing in Brooklyn.

- Catch the B82 bus, bound for Starrett/Spring Creek, on the south side of Kings Hwy. While waiting, note the crown decorations hanging from the street lamps—crowns on Kings (they're illuminated at night). This was purportedly the first U.S. road designated a highway. It connected the original settlements of Kings County and is more properly, and Britishly, called *the* Kings Hwy.

- Get off the bus at E. 22nd St. Immediately south of Kings Hwy. on E. 22nd is the Wyckoff-Bennett home. Its year of construction is pegged at 1766, based on an engraving in one of its wood beams. The farm it was built for extended all the way south to the ocean, and after the city adopted a street grid the house had to be moved 90 degrees to face west instead of south.

- Proceed south on E. 22nd. This is one of those areas of Brooklyn with no definitive affiliation. You're east of Gravesend and north of Sheepshead Bay, though I'm sure you could find people who would group it with one or the other. If you define a neighborhood by its people, you'd consider it Midwood because of the Orthodox Jews, but Kings Hwy. has historically been considered the southern boundary of Midwood. Still others cling to virtually obsolete monikers like Homecrest and Madison, from when these communities were first developed residentially. Regardless, it's a pleasant place for a tranquil walk amid nicely maintained if not historically significant houses.

- Turn right on Avenue R. This area was much rowdier about 100 years ago, when two immensely popular racetracks were in business. They were shut down when New York State enacted an antibetting law around 1910.

- Turn left on Ocean Pkwy. so you can experience a snippet of this landscaped boulevard created by Frederick Law Olmsted and Calvert Vaux in their Prospect Park design. They planned this and Eastern Pkwy. with grassy malls, trees, and pedestrian paths to extend nature from the park out into the city.

- Turn right on Gravesend Neck Rd., also called just Neck Rd. Trinity Tabernacle, a gospel church, stands on your right past Avenue V. Its building was constructed in 1893 as the third house of worship for a Dutch Reformed congregation founded in 1655. The Victorian parsonage next to the church dates to 1901.

- When you cross Village Rd. E., you're within the bounds of the original town of Gravesend. Lady Moody was a visionary of urban planning as well as sociopolitics. She laid out four quadrants, each with an equal number of lots and a commons at the center—a design regarded as a forerunner of modern urban planning. Gravesend Neck Rd. was the village's east-west road, McDonald Ave. (then Gravesend Ave.) the north-south artery. The house at #27, on your right after McDonald, sits on the lots owned by Lady Moody. She may or may not have lived in this particular house, which was built sometime in the 17th century. It is one of Brooklyn's oldest houses, and some are irked by the later addition of fluted columns and a faux stone exterior uncharacteristic of its period. Across the street are two cemeteries where Gravesend's original settlers and American Revolution soldiers were interred, though virtually all the 17th-century headstones have crumbled away or are illegible. You wouldn't have been able to identify Lady Moody's grave anyway—it was unmarked.

- Turn right on Van Sicklen St., which took its name from one of Brooklyn's first and wealthiest Dutch families. The public school here was built around 1913, in a dramatic style known as Collegiate Gothic that includes a terra cotta parapet with open quatrefoils and gargoyles. The fabulous Victorian house across from the school dates to the 1860s and initially belonged to someone in the Van Strycker family, another of Brooklyn's early power brokers.

- Turn right on Village Rd. N. and walk into Lady Moody Triangle. After looking at its granite monument memorializing World War II and the founding of Gravesend, pick up a pastry at Nuccio's across Avenue U, a main commercial thoroughfare of southern Brooklyn and a good place for ethnic snacking. Farther east, there are Chinese and Russian eateries; here, the flavor tends to be Italian.

- Cross back to Village Rd. N., the northern boundary in Lady Moody's town design, and go left. The house at #32 was built around 1788 as a school (which George Washington once visited) and was later used as Gravesend's town hall in the 1800s. Next to it, #38 is a Dutch Colonial from the mid-1800s, known as the Ryder-Van Cleef House.

- Cross over back to Avenue U and go right. Turn left on E. 2nd, then left on Avenue T. You'll see some of the big new residences that are altering the look of this historic neighborhood. Then turn right on McDonald Ave. A nursing home, basketball courts, an auto body shop, a huge yeshiva, and the elevated train surround Hubbard House, built around 1770. It may look like it's fighting for its life amid all these 20th-century encroachments, but the mortgage was financed through the New York Landmarks Conservancy, which should protect it. The taller wing was added in the 1920s.

- Continue on McDonald to the other side of Avenue S for the subway.

*Old Gravesend Cemetery*

## Caring For Caruso

Aldo Mancusi, a retired contractor who has lived in Brooklyn his whole life, inherited a love of music from his parents, who played the piano and sang. He also inherited his father's record collection, which was heavy on Enrico Caruso. About 35 years ago Mancusi started collecting on his own, not just recordings but photos, programs, personal effects, and other memorabilia related to the illustrious Italian tenor. Today, Mancusi runs the Enrico Caruso Museum of America on the top floor of his home on E. 19th St., between Avenues S and T. No place in Italy has such an extensive Caruso collection, and Mancusi's work has earned him an honorary title, *cavaliere ufficiale*, from the Italian government. Among the more unusual items displayed are a canceled check signed by Caruso, Mardi Gras tokens and novelty dollar bills with his likeness on them, "Caruso recipes" that were inserted in pasta boxes, a death mask, and many caricatures drawn by Caruso (a sketch artist on the side). The museum also contains antique instruments and costumes and scenery pieces from the Metropolitan Opera donated by soprano Licia Albanese. There's even a 12-seat theater. Call 718-368-3993 to visit by appointment or to attend one of Mancusi's lecture/tours, which usually include a film screening. Go to www.enricocarusomuseum.com for more information.

## POINTS OF INTEREST

**Wyckoff-Bennett Homestead** 1669 E. 22nd St., Brooklyn, NY 11229

**Lady Moody's House** 27 Gravesend Neck Rd., Brooklyn, NY 11223

**Lady Moody Triangle** Van Sicklen St. between Avenue U and Village Rd. N., Brooklyn, NY 11223

**Nuccio's** 261 Avenue U, Brooklyn, NY 11223, 718-449-3035

**Ryder-Van Cleef House** 38 Village Rd. N., Brooklyn, NY 11223

**Hubbard House** 2138 McDonald Ave., Brooklyn, NY 11223

# route summary

1.  Begin at Kings Hwy. and E. 22nd St. and walk south on E. 22nd.

2.  Turn right on Avenue R.

3.  Turn left on Ocean Pkwy.

4.  Turn right on Gravesend Neck Rd.

5.  Turn right on Van Sicklen St.

6.  Turn right at Village Rd. N. for Lady Moody Triangle.

7.  Cross back to Village Rd. N. and then to Avenue U and go right. Then turn left on E. 2nd St., left on Avenue T, and right on McDonald Ave. to Hubbard House.

8.  Continue on McDonald to the Kings Hwy. F train station.

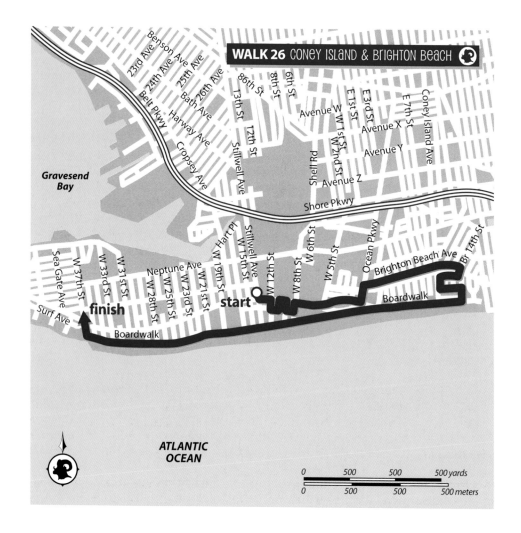

**WALK 26** CONEY ISLAND & BRIGHTON BEACH

Gravesend
Bay

23rd Ave
Benson Ave
24th Ave
25th Ave
26th Ave
Bath Ave
Belt Pkwy
Harway Ave
Cropsey Ave
13th St
12th St
Stillwell Ave
86th St
8th St
6th St
Avenue W
W 1st St
W 2nd St
E 1st St
E 3rd St
E 7th St
Avenue X
Avenue Y
Shell Rd
Avenue Z
Coney Island Ave
Shore Pkwy

Sea Gate Ave
W 37th St
W 33rd St
W 31st St
W 28th St
W 25th St
W 23rd St
W 21st St
W 19th St
Hart Pl
Stillwell Ave
W 15th St
W 12th St
W 8th St
W 6th St
W 5th St
Ocean Pkwy
Brighton Beach Ave
Br 12th St

Neptune Ave

**finish**
Surf Ave
Boardwalk

**start**
Boardwalk

ATLANTIC
OCEAN

0    500    500    500 yards
0    500    500    500 meters

# 26 CONEY ISLAND AND BRIGHTON BEACH: OLD TIMES AND OLD WORLD ON THE BOARDWALK

**BOUNDARIES:** Boardwalk, Seacoast Terr., Brighton Beach Ave., W. 37th St.
**DISTANCE:** Approx. 4 miles
**SUBWAY:** D, F, N, or Q to Stillwell Ave.

Long before Vegas and Orlando, Coney Island was America's playground. And by the time places like Vegas and Orlando were booming, Coney Island—the progenitor of every theme-park destination and beach resort across the land—was in serious decline. But sometime in the 1990s the inklings of a revival took hold. Since then, millions of dollars have been poured into the neighborhood: a pro baseball stadium was built, then new music and changing pavilions on the Boardwalk, and ultimately a showplace-caliber subway station. This walk covers the neighborhood of Coney Island and three-quarters of the island of Coney itself (really more of a peninsula since a 1910 landfilling), including all three miles of the famous Boardwalk.

- Exit the subway station on Stillwell Ave. and cross the street to take a gander at the mural that looks like a collaboration between Lewis Carroll and Joan Miró. Facing the mural, go to your left. Those rusty painted posts at every corner of Stillwell and Surf Aves. were electrification poles for the trolleys. The corner building on your right dates to the 1920s and has held onto the neon vertical signage from its days as the Shore theater.

- Cross Surf to Nathan's, dispenser of top dogs (their fries are awesome too). The hot dog was invented in Coney Island when Feltman's restaurant put German sausages inside elongated buns. Feltman's employee Nathan Handwerker took the "recipe" and started selling franks for 5¢ apiece—half what Feltman's charged—at his own stand in 1916. Nathan's is now a fast-food franchise, but this is the one and only original.

- From Nathan's, take a moment to examine the subway station where you arrived. The BMT tiles on Surf Ave. were salvaged from the original station built here in the 1920s, and the pyramidal roof resembles a structure from Coney's old Steeplechase amusement park. When Coney Island first developed as a vacation resort in the 1870s, it catered to the middle and upper classes; the opening of a subway station here around 1920 made it accessible to the working class, and on summer weekends in the 1920s and '30s a million people a day streamed through the turnstiles.

- Cross Stillwell. Relics on this block include the Surf Hotel sign on the corner building and the former Henderson's music hall—now recognizable merely as the tallest yellow building down Stillwell to your right. Head east on Surf past two vintage façades: Faber's Fascination, which was a bingo hall, and Herman Popper & Bro., a distillery/saloon. The stateliness of the 1904 Popper building is easy to overlook amid the surrounding rigmarole. Eldorado Auto Skooter next door is itself housed in a Greek Revival structure (disco effects added later). A couple of doors farther, visit the Coney Island Museum upstairs at 1208 Surf Ave. for a neighborhood history lesson replete with funhouse mirrors and other memorabilia. Every year on the first Saturday after the summer solstice, the Mardi Gra-esque Mermaid Parade frolics down Surf Ave.

- Turn right on W. 12th St. The Coney Island renaissance aims not to sanitize but to preserve and honor the past, even when that means bringing back such dubious entertainments as the freak show . . . which is here on your right at Sideshows by the Seashore, in a 1917 restaurant building.

- Turn left on Bowery St., created as a passageway in 1898 to the then-new Steeplechase Park and named after the similarly honky-tonk Manhattan street. Beside the Wonder Wheel Thrills sign, the white building with two chimneylike projections is all that's left of Feltman's restaurant.

- Turn left on Jones Walk, pausing to drop a quarter in the mechanized diorama of Coney Island, or in the chimp's head if you prefer. These are small-scale examples of the nostalgia-driven renaissance that's bringing in new versions of old-time amusements.

- Back at Surf Ave., you're facing a furniture store on the site of the entrance to Luna Park, the largest of Coney Island's fantasy worlds, filled with minarets, spires, and domes for a skyline modeled after Baghdad. Luna shut down in 1944. Its most famous rides provided "trips" to the moon and the North Pole.

- Turn right on W. 10th St., aka Dewey Albert Pl. after the man who founded Astroland and had the Cyclone restored. And there the landmark roller coaster is on your left.

It's been rattling daredevil riders over 12 drops in two minutes since 1927, when it took the place of the Switchback Railway (1884), the world's first roller coaster. On the other side of W. 10th, the Coney Island Hall of Fame is a wall of tributes to the impresarios and businessmen whose legacies we explore on this walk.

● Return to Surf and turn right. The New York Aquarium on your right is on the site of Dreamland, the fantastic amusement park lost to a 1911 fire after only seven years in business. Ironically, one of its top attractions was a fire rescue simulation. European artwork, landmarks, and scenery were replicated inside the park. Continue on Surf into Brighton Beach, which also developed as a seaside resort in the late 1800s and is now Russian through and through. Cross the avenue at W. 5th St. Walk on Surf alongside Asser Levy Park a short distance, entering the park where some benches and bushes encircle a trilevel round planter, a memorial to the Russian-American victims of 9/11.

● Staying in the park, leave the memorial area via the path to your left. Follow it past a playground, a large lawn, and the bandshell to a park exit on Seabreeze Ave.

● Go left on Ocean Pkwy., then turn right beneath the viaduct onto Brighton Beach Ave. This is a great place for noshing, with shops and restaurants that sell baked goods on the sidewalk and several produce stands too. You may want to put together a meal at M&I International, the largest Russian supermarket in town (between Brighton 1st Pl. and 2nd St.). It has a deli counter, bakery, butcher, and a vast selection of packaged goods from many countries. In the back, hot entrees and homemade Russian specialties are sold by the pound. For a

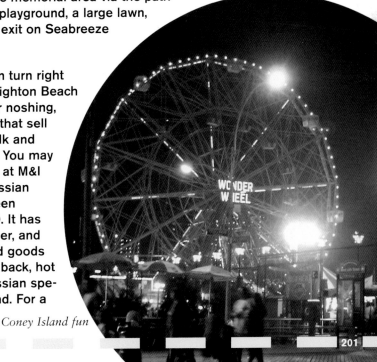

*Coney Island fun*

sit-down meal, area restaurants serve cuisine not just from Russia but from other former Soviet republics and their neighbors—for instance, Primorski (between 2nd and 3rd) is Georgian, and Kashkar Café (down at 14th) is run by Uygurs, Muslims from western China. Restaurants such as National, Atlantic Oceana, and Odessa feature dinner banquets and ingratiatingly cheesy revues.

- To your right at Coney Island Ave. is one of the largest and most controversial real-estate developments in all of Brooklyn, the Oceana condominiums. Some have objected to the Florida-like complex being laid down in New York City. Even more opposition has come from those who didn't like seeing Brighton Beach's most famous destination erased. The Brighton Beach Bath and Racquet Club stood here from 1919 into the 21st century. In its heyday, celebrities were on the guest register as well as on the stages performing. Tilyou Playground, a pleasant public green space on Brighton Beach Ave. between 11th and 13th Sts., is an Oceana peace offering to the community. Walk a little farther east and you'll see that history has not been completely eradicated: at 14th and 15th Sts., Art Deco apartment houses remain.

- Go back to Coney Island Ave. and turn left. Enter the Oceana complex on your left to walk around and see for yourself what the fuss is about. Exit on Seacoast Terr., straight across from where you came in.

- Turn right on Seacoast Terr., then right onto the Boardwalk. Even in summer, this section of beach is much mellower than Coney's. About 1,000 feet along, you'll find a string of Russian restaurants that offer open-air dining and a distinctly Old World ambience. This is where Little Odessa most resembles the Black Sea town in its nickname.

- At Ocean Pkwy., cross back into Coney Island. Next to the New York Aquarium is Astroland. The amusement park is slated to close after the 2007 season, and luxury condos, a hotel, and new rides are planned for the future. But resistance to this plan for a year-round resort could keep Astroland around longer. Regardless, the Cyclone will stay.

- Next comes Deno's Amusement Park. The horses in the carousel are not authentic wooden oldies, but they're known as Coney Island horses because of their pastel

*A summer's day at Coney Island*

colors. Walk through the tunnel beside the carousel to reach the Wonder Wheel. This Ferris wheel dates to 1920, but one of the oldest things in all of Coney Island is in the arcade opposite its ticket booth: Grandma's Predictions, located immediately on your right. She's been telling fortunes since around 1900, and she breathes—watch her chest if you splurge on the quarter.

- Return to the Boardwalk and resume your walk west. Go into Ruby's Bar & Grill for its museum-like display of old pictures. After Ruby's, there's a Shoot the Freak booth—more benign than it sounds. It's merely a paintball game with one not-so-freakily costumed human being among the targets. (Both Ruby's and Shoot the Freak may close for redevelopment.) From the Boardwalk at Stillwell, the land mass you see across the water is the shore town of Sandy Hook, New Jersey.

- Your next turn off the Boardwalk will be to the left—onto 1,000-foot-long Steeplechase Pier. Walk to the end and turn around for the ultimate Coney Island panorama. Opposite the pier on the Boardwalk rises the 277-foot Parachute Jump, which was erected for the 1939 World's Fair (held in Queens) and moved to Coney in 1941. It was refurbished in 2006 as a beacon—outfitted with 17 flood lamps, 150 light fixtures, and 450 LEDs and illuminated nightly in varying patterns, including one that mimics the waxing and waning of the moon.

- A sign below the Parachute Jump tells you this is the former site of Steeplechase Park, the longest-lived of Coney Island's legendary amusement parks. Steeplechase launched Coney Island's amusement-park heyday and managed to stay open until 1964. Today there's another kind of park here—KeySpan Park, home field of the minor-league Brooklyn Cyclones, who brought professional baseball back to Brooklyn in 2001, 44 years after the Dodgers' defection. The Thunderbolt roller coaster once stood in the field next to the ballpark. It was the world's first steel-framed roller coaster and was featured in Woody Allen's childhood flashback in *Annie Hall*—he blamed his neuroses on growing up in a house beneath the roller coaster (yes, there actually was a house under the Thunderbolt).

- As you continue west on the Boardwalk, the next landmark (just past 21st St.) is unmissable—long-shuttered Child's restaurant, built in 1924 and justly renowned for its terra cotta decorations of ships and sea creatures. Has anything this decrepit ever looked so great? This was the "Coney Island Community Center" that Sandra Bullock was trying to save in *Two Weeks Notice.*

- You're now leaving Coney Island's central business (or pleasure) district. Many visitors don't bother with the Boardwalk beyond it, so you should feel like an explorer— which would be apt, since Henry Hudson landed right around here back in 1609. The white apartment building between 28th and 29th Sts. replaced the Half Moon Hotel (named after Hudson's ship), which welcomed guests from the turn of the century into the 1950s.

- The Boardwalk becomes much more tranquil as you proceed west. Look for the nautical-themed playground past 29th St. Soon after that, cruise ships sailing out of Red Hook might look awfully close.

- When the Boardwalk ends at W. 37th St., go back onto Surf Ave. The island extends another ½ mile, but access is restricted to residents and guests of Sea Gate, a private but not especially posh gated community. Before Sea Gate became an exclusive community around 1900, it was a seedy district of dance halls, gambling dens, and brothels.

- Cross Surf Ave. to take the B36 bus back to the Stillwell Ave. subway. (Get the bus on the westbound side of the street even though you want to go east.)

# POINTS OF INTEREST

**Nathan's** Surf and Stillwell Aves., Brooklyn, NY 11224, 718-946-2202
**Coney Island Museum** 1208 Surf Ave., Brooklyn, NY 11224, 718-372-5159
**Sideshows by the Seashore** 3006 W. 12th St., Brooklyn, NY 11224, 718-372-5159
**New York Aquarium** W. 8th St. and Surf Ave., Brooklyn, NY 11224, 718-265-FISH
**Asser Levy Park** W. 5th St. between Surf and Seaview Aves., Brooklyn, NY 11224
**M&I International** 249 Brighton Beach Ave., Brooklyn, NY 11235, 718-615-1011
**Primorski** 282 Brighton Beach Ave., Brooklyn, NY 11235, 718-891-3111
**Kashkar Café** 1141 Brighton Beach Ave., Brooklyn, NY 11235, 718-743-3832
**Tilyou Playground** Brighton Beach Ave. between 11th and 13th Sts., Brooklyn, NY 11224
**Astroland Amusement Park** Coney Island Boardwalk at W. 10th St., Brooklyn, NY 11224, 718-265-2100
**Deno's Amusement Park** Coney Island Boardwalk at W. 12th St., Brooklyn, NY 11224, 718-372-2592

# ROUTE SUMMARY

1. Begin at Surf and Stillwell Aves. and go east on Surf.
2. Turn right on W. 12th St.
3. Turn left on Bowery St.
4. Turn left on Jones Walk.
5. Turn right on Surf.
6. Turn right on W. 10th St., then go back to Surf and go right.
7. Walk through Asser Levy Park, exiting at Seabreeze Ave.
8. Turn left on Ocean Pkwy., then right on Brighton Beach Ave.
9. At 15th St., turn around and go back to Coney Island Ave. and go left.
10. Walk through Oceana to Seacoast Terr. and turn right.
11. Turn right on the Boardwalk.
12. Turn right on W. 37th St. and get the bus at Surf Ave.

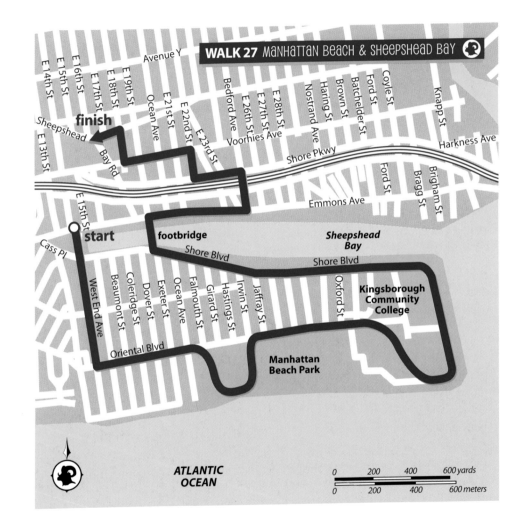

**WALK 27** Manhattan Beach & Sheepshead Bay

E 14th St
E 15th St
E 16th St
E 17th St
E 18th St
E 19th St

Avenue Y

Sheepshead

**finish**

E 13th St

Bay Rd

E 21st St
E 22nd St
E 23rd St

Ocean Ave

Bedford Ave
E 26th St
E 27th St
E 28th St

Voorhies Ave

Nostrand Ave
Haring St
Brown St
Batchelder St
Ford St
Coyle St

Knapp St

Harkness Ave

Shore Pkwy

Ford St
Bragg St
Brigham St

Emmons Ave

E 15th St

**start**

Cass Pl

West End Ave

**footbridge**

Shore Blvd

Beaumont St
Coleridge St
Dover St
Exeter St
Ocean Ave
Falmouth St
Girard St
Hastings St
Irwin St
Jaffray St

Shore Blvd

Oxford St

*Sheepshead Bay*

**Kingsborough Community College**

Oriental Blvd

**Manhattan Beach Park**

*ATLANTIC OCEAN*

0    200    400    600 yards
0    200    400    600 meters

# 27 Manhattan Beach and Sheepshead Bay: Finery and Fishery at the Coast

BOUNDARIES: **West End Ave., Oriental Blvd., Kingsborough Community College, Jerome Ave.**
DISTANCE: **Approx. 4¼ miles**
SUBWAY: **B or Q to Sheepshead Bay, transfer to B49 bus to Kingsborough Community College**

Like their western neighbors Coney Island and Brighton Beach, Manhattan Beach and Sheepshead Bay first developed as vacation destinations, albeit with distinct identities. Manhattan Beach was upscale, Sheepshead Bay a more down-to-earth bungalow colony. In Manhattan Beach, affluent hotel guests gave way to affluent homeowners, who continue to build bigger and fancier today. Meanwhile, construction of condos and townhouses around Sheepshead Bay is altering the look of its waterfront and diminishing its resemblance to a New England fishing village. Still, that old-time charm and seafaring industry thrive here more than anywhere else in Brooklyn.

● Get off the bus at Emmons Ave. and Shore Blvd. Here at the border between Sheepshead Bay and Manhattan Beach, abutting the marina, is Holocaust Memorial Park. This was the first public Holocaust memorial established in New York City, and the site was chosen partly because of the area's sizable Jewish population. Ironically, Manhattan Beach was developed by an avowed anti-Semite. Austin Corbin, a lawyer and financier—and member of the American Society for the Suppression of Jews— transformed a rural spit known as Sedge Bank into the swanky resort of Manhattan Beach with his hotels and railroad. One block over, a street named Corbin Pl. straddles the border between Manhattan Beach and Brighton Beach, home to many Jews of Russian descent.

● Cross Shore Blvd. and walk south on West End Ave. The boarded-up kiosk at West End and Oriental Blvd. is a 100-year-old remnant from Manhattan Beach's days as a gated community. The angular house just off Oriental Blvd. at 219 West End Ave. was designed by architect Arkady Zaltsman, a Brooklyn resident from Moldova who was meeting with a client on the 105th floor of the World Trade Center on 9/11. He died at age 45.

- Walk east on Oriental Blvd., but feel free to detour in and out of side streets to see other opulent homes. Many streets have British names—a common conceit among real-estate developers in the early 20th century. The exception is Ocean Ave., which extends far beyond Manhattan Beach.

- At Falmouth St., enter Manhattan Beach Park. Meander around the park and find your way to the beach. This most secluded, most tranquil of New York City's beaches has not been discovered by many people outside the neighborhood. Once upon a time, however, nearly everyone in New York knew about this spot—which corresponds approximately to the location of Austin Corbin's extravagant Manhattan Beach and Oriental hotels. President Ulysses S. Grant cut the ribbon at the Manhattan Beach's opening in 1877, and his successor, Rutherford B. Hayes, would do the same when the larger, more expensive Oriental was dedicated in 1880. Circus performances and historic reenactments were held at the hotels, as well as concerts conducted by the likes of Victor Herbert and John Philip Sousa, who premiered "Stars and Stripes Forever" in Manhattan Beach.

- Head back to Oriental at Irwin St. and go right. The park runs all the way to Mackenzie St. Canine lovers may want to pause at the dog run between Jaffray and Kensington Sts. On the opposite side of Oriental, check out the old houses near Norfolk, including #1605 with its observation deck.

- Continue east on Oriental Blvd. and into Kingsborough Community College. After passing the security booth, go right and walk through a couple of parking lots to get to the college's own beach. Follow the water's edge all the way around campus. You're tracing the eastern perimeter of Coney Island. The view includes the Marine Parkway Gil Hodges Memorial Bridge, which links Brooklyn with Queens' Rockaway peninsula, and Plumb Beach, part of Gateway National Recreation Area. This scenic campus belongs to a 40-year-old junior college run by the city, and one of its academic buildings doubles as a lighthouse.

- Leave the campus through its north gate, which puts you on Shore Blvd. Walk beside the Sheepshead Bay marina. Try to spot the old bungalows that have survived amid the mansionizing of Shore Blvd. The handsome building with the cupola to your left on Irwin is P.S. 195, ranked as one of New York City's best elementary schools.

- At Exeter St., cross the marina via the wooden footbridge that has spanned this waterway since 1882. It too was built by Corbin. When you step off the bridge in Sheepshead Bay, you're opposite Lundy's Landing. This mall contains shops, offices, and eateries, but for many years the entire space was occupied by one restaurant. Lundy's had started on a pier in 1916 and opened in this Spanish Mission–style building—now a city landmark—in 1934 as the largest restaurant in the country. It could seat 2,800 customers, many of whom dined on a five-course surf-and-turf "shore dinner" that still cost less than $20 when the place closed in 1979. A later incarnation, less than a third the size of the original, operated under different owners from 1995 to 2007.

- Turn right on Emmons Ave., which used to be lined with seafood restaurants. Now the menus vary from Asian to Slavic to Mediterranean and more. You may want to stop for a coffee or pastry at the Turkish-run Masal Cafe in the Lundy's building. One veteran still drawing seafood fans is Randazzo's at E. 21st St. Those who prefer to cook their own come to the Sheepshead docks, just east of Randazzo's, around four o'clock to buy the day's catch right off a boat. The house at 2235 Emmons Ave., near Dooley St., is the sole survivor of a group of elegant vacation homes built around 1870.

- Turn left on Bedford Ave., the longest road in Brooklyn (it runs more than 10 miles from Emmons Ave. north to Williamsburg).

- Go left on Shore Pkwy., then right on E. 22nd St. Kenmore Ct. on your left, with its alley of bungalow homes, provides a glimpse of old Sheepshead.

- From E. 22nd, turn left on Voorhies Ave. A number of architectural eras

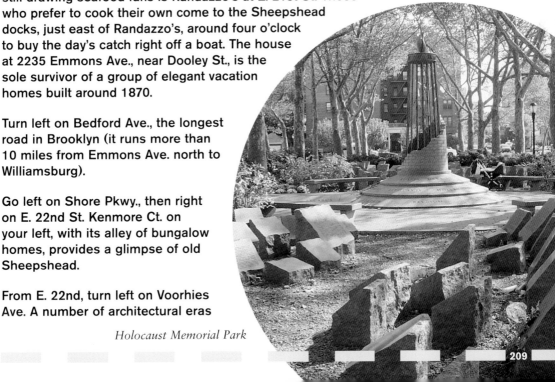

*Holocaust Memorial Park*

and genres converge at Voorhies and Ocean Aves. The Methodist church on your left has been here since 1869. It shares the intersection with an Art Deco apartment house, a boxy modern apartment building, and a strip mall. Farther along Voorhies between E. 19th and E. 18th Sts. are a couple of vintage homes.

● Turn right on E. 18th St. At Jerome Ave., the campanile you can see to your right is part of a church named St. Mark's—just like the piazza in Venice with the campanile this one obviously copies. Go left on Jerome.

● Before entering the B/Q subway station on your left at E. 15th St., turn right to see the mural beneath the train trestle, which portrays Sheepshead Bay from the days of cobblestone lanes and trolleys to a contemporary streetscape of Rollerbladers and fast food. The wooden bridge you walked on is depicted too. There are also ceramic-tile murals of Sheepshead history in the train station—look for the fish pattern within them.

## POINTS OF INTEREST

**Holocaust Memorial Park** Shore Blvd. and Emmons Ave., Brooklyn, NY 11235, 718-743-3636

**Manhattan Beach Park** Oriental Blvd. between Ocean Ave. and Mackenzie St., Brooklyn, NY 11235

**Kingsborough Community College** 2001 Oriental Blvd., Brooklyn, NY 11235, 718-265-5343

**Masal Cafe** 1901 Emmons Ave., Brooklyn, NY 11235, 718-891-7090

**Randazzo's** 2017 Emmons Ave., Brooklyn, NY 11235, 718-615-0010

# route summary

1. Take the B49 bus to Holocaust Memorial Park at Emmons Ave. and Shore Blvd.

2. Cross Shore Blvd. and walk south on West End Ave.

3. Turn left on Oriental Blvd.

4. Enter Manhattan Beach Park at Falmouth St. Exit at Irwin St. and resume walking east on Oriental to reach Kingsborough Community College.

5. Walk around the campus to Shore Blvd.

6. Cross the wooden bridge from Exeter St.

7. Turn right on Emmons Ave.

8. Turn left on Bedford Ave.

9. Turn left on Shore Pkwy., then right on E. 22nd St.

10. Turn left on Voorhies Ave.

11. Turn right on E. 18th St., then left on Jerome Ave.

12. Board the B or Q subway at Jerome and E. 15th St.

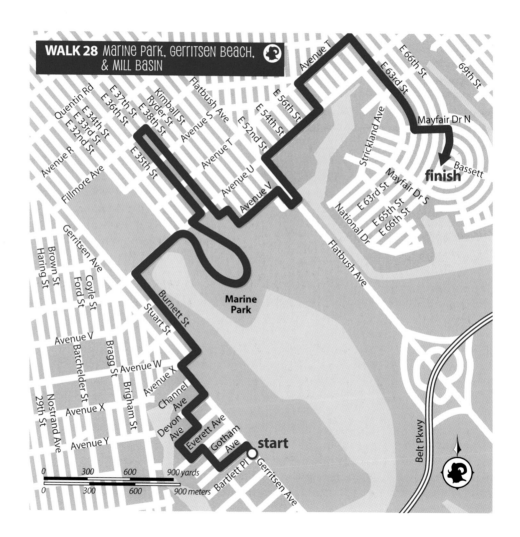

WALK 28 Marine Park, Gerritsen Beach, & Mill Basin

Quentin Rd
E 37th St
E 34th St
E 33rd St
E 32nd St
Kimball St
Ryder St
E 38th St
E 36th St
E 35th St
Avenue S
Avenue R
Flatbush Ave
Fillmore Ave

Avenue T
E 56th St
E 54th St
E 52nd St
Avenue T
Avenue S

Avenue T
Avenue U
Avenue V

E 66th St
E 63rd St
69th St
Mayfair Dr N
Strickland Ave
Mayfair Dr S
E 63rd St
E 65th St
E 66th St
National Dr
Bassett

**finish**

Flatbush Ave

Gerritsen Ave
Brown St
Haring St
Coyle St
Ford St
Burnett St
Stuart St

**Marine Park**

Avenue V
Avenue W
Avenue X
Avenue X
Avenue Y
Batchelder St
Bragg St
Brigham St
Nostrand Ave
29th St
Channel Ave
Devon Ave
Everett Ave
Gotham Ave
Bartlett Pl
Gerritsen Ave

**start**

Belt Pkwy

0    300    600    900 yards
0    300    600    900 meters

# 28 Marine Park, Gerritsen Beach, and Mill Basin: Nautical and Natural

BOUNDARIES: **Bartlett Pl., Joval Ct., Fillmore Ave., E. 58th or E. 63rd St.**
DISTANCE: **Approx. 5 or 6¼ miles, depending on route chosen**
SUBWAY: **B or Q to Kings Hwy., transfer to B31 bus to Gerritsen Beach**

Marine Park, Gerritsen Beach, Mill Basin . . . these are places unfamiliar to a lot of New Yorkers. Located on a peninsula of southeastern Brooklyn, unserved by the subway, these are traditional, family-oriented communities with a nautical vibe and, in some places, a degree of affluence. They border the Rockaway Inlet of Jamaica Bay, and a number of channels and creeks cut into the land. A chunk of the region lies within the Gateway National Recreation Area (26,600 waterfront acres encompassing parts of Brooklyn, Queens, Staten Island, and New Jersey), including Marine Park—Brooklyn's largest park—namesake of the neighborhood, and home to a wetland habitat for crustaceans, mollusks, and over 100 bird species.

- Get off the bus on Gerritsen Ave. at Bartlett Pl., in front of the Gerritsen Beach branch of the public library. Go inside if the library's open and walk toward the back, where a picture window looks out on Shell Bank Canal.

- Upon exiting the library, go to your left on Gerritsen Ave., then turn left on Gotham Ave. You're walking past the houses with backyard docks that you saw from the library. Peek between the houses at Shell Bank Canal, which was created by the real-estate entrepreneur who developed Gerritsen Beach as a summer bungalow colony in the 1920s.

- Turn right on Fane Ct. On both sides of the canal, the north-south streets are alphabetically named courts; on this side, the east-west avenues are also alphabetical. The streets are quite uniform—bungalow-type houses close together on small lots without front yards. Combined with the sea air, you've got a picture-postcard fishing village.

- Turn left on Everett Ave., then right on Joval Ct. At the water's edge at Devon Ave., you'll find what you always expect to see at a marina . . . horses! A nearby homeowner, who hires out horses for weddings and special events, keeps a stable here.

- After visiting with the horses, proceed on Devon Ave. to Ebony Ct. and turn left. It leads right into the Tamaqua Marina, which has been in existence more than 70 years under the same family's ownership. The bar and restaurant are open to the public.

- From the marina, walk on Channel Ave. to Gerritsen Ave. and turn left. Walk on the right side of Gerritsen, following the sidewalk past P.S. 277 and through Dr. John's Playground. Dr. John Elefterakis, who suffered a fatal brain aneurysm at age 37, was a P.S. 277 alumnus who returned to Gerritsen Beach to practice medicine. He was also medical director of the Vollies—Brooklyn's only volunteer fire department, which has served Gerritsen Beach since 1921.

- Turn right on Christopher Columbus Dr., aka Avenue X, then turn left on Burnett St. You're walking alongside Marine Park Creek and its salt marsh. From the VFW memorial at Whitney Ave., you can see across the creek to the salt marsh and nature center you'll be visiting in a while. Continue on Burnett, which at the turn of the century was the site of a 65-acre horseracing estate. Much of the property was donated to the city in 1920 and formed the basis of Marine Park.

- Turn right on Avenue U. The recreational fields of Marine Park are on your left, and people may be fishing in the creek on your right. White Island (Mau Mau to locals), a city dump turned bird sanctuary, is in the middle of the creek. At 798 acres, Marine Park ranks seventh in size in New York City, and its most valuable asset is the natural habitat of the salt marsh, whose ecosystem acts as a water purifier and erosion barrier. You can learn all about it on the 1-mile trail through the marsh, which begins at the nature center on your right at E. 33rd St. Be sure to read the first marker on the route about the 17th-century gristmill. Wherever the trail offers two paths, go to your right, except toward the end after the RESIDENTS AND VISITORS: BIRDS AT MARINE PARK sign. Before or after walking the trail, go inside the nature center for more informative exhibits.

- When you leave the nature center area, go right on Avenue U. Go left on E. 36th St. for a stroll through residential Marine Park. Homeowners here seem to enjoy exterior decorating, and some have beautiful flower gardens in season. One of the city's oldest houses is on your left past Avenue S: Hendrick I. Lott House, a structure with landmark status that may eventually be open to the public. Its east wing was constructed in 1720, the rest of it in 1800. Brooklyn College has been doing archaeological excavations on the grounds since 1997 and has unearthed West African artifacts (presumably owned by slaves) along with Lott family possessions.

- Turn right on Fillmore Ave., then right on E. 37th St. Back at Avenue U, proceed into Lenape Playground, named for the native inhabitants of this area. Their totem poles are replicated in the park, which also features oversize snake and tortoise sculptures where kids can climb and play.

- Exit the playground at E. 38th St. and go right. Then go left on Avenue V. The Marine Park Golf Course is on your right, beyond the trees.

- At Flatbush Ave., cross over and turn right. You have a better view of the golf course to your right, but the more interesting sight is on your left. Go just past Hendrickson Pl. to see the marina in back of Kings Plaza shopping center. The body of water is Mill Basin; the neighborhood across the water is Mill Island, the ritzy part of the neighborhood named Mill Basin.

- Walk back in the direction you came on Flatbush Ave. and turn right on Avenue U, which, believe it or not, used to be a stream. Continue past Kings Plaza (Brooklyn's first mall) to

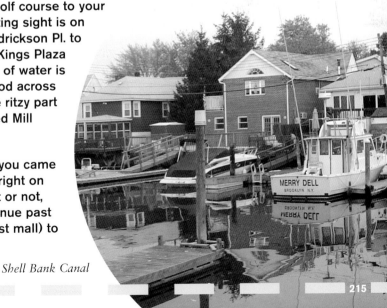

*Shell Bank Canal*

local dining favorites—the food stands at E. 58th St. If you're here in warmer months, you definitely want to try one or two of the 60-plus flavors at Dolly's Ices. Food is also available if you continue to Mill Basin. But you can end your walk here by taking the westbound B3 bus on Avenue U and transferring to the Q train at E. 16th St.

Addendum:

- Turn left onto E. 58th St. and turn right at Avenue T for Mill Basin Kosher Deli and Art Gallery. As the *Mona Lisa* is to the Louvre, works by Erté are to this restaurant. Its owner is a foremost collector and dealer of works by the Art Deco master, who reportedly visited the deli late in his life and designed its awning. As for what's on the tables rather than the walls, it's one of the best places in the five boroughs for Jewish deli food, one of NYC's indigenous cuisines.

- Continue going northeast on Avenue T. The oldest dwellings around here were built between the 1920s and '40s, narrow frame houses on 20-by-100-foot lots. The wider old houses date to the late 1940s and early '50s, when lots had expanded to 50-by-100. The houses are essentially identical: go a few steps to your right down, say, Mill Ave. and look at the symmetry of chimneys at the backs of the Avenue T houses.

- From Avenue T, turn right onto E. 63rd St. Since the 1980s, many original homes of Mill Basin have been razed to make room for custom-built manses. Back in the 1950s, the Brooklyn Museum took care of a true neighborhood original—the Jan Martense Schenck House, built in 1675—by dismantling it and later reassembling it inside the museum. It can still be visited there. Schenck's house was located here on E. 63rd, south of what is now Strickland Ave. After Strickland, you have crossed from Mill Basin into Mill Island, where families live in luxury on land where 17th- and 18th-century farmers erected grain mills powered by the tides of Jamaica Bay.

- Turn left on Mayfair Dr. N. and right on E. 66th St. The house at the southeast corner is one of the most extravagant in the neighborhood. Another eyepopper, pink with tall arched windows, is just off E. 66th on Gaylord Dr.

- Conclude your walk at E. 66th and Bassett Ave., in front of the multi-iron-gated behemoth with dual staircases. You have three options from here. If it's a weekday, just wait for the Midwood-bound B100 and take it to the B/Q subway at Kings Hwy.

That bus runs only every half hour on Saturday and every hour on Sunday, so on weekends you may prefer to walk back to Avenue U for the westbound B3 and then transfer to the Q train at E. 16th St. Your third choice, if you still have leg power, is to meander through more of Mill Island's concentric-circle streets. The most expensive properties are waterside on National Dr. and Indiana Pl.

## POINTS OF INTEREST

**Brooklyn Public Library–Gerritsen Beach** 2808 Gerritsen Ave., Brooklyn, NY 11229, 718-368-1435

**Tamaqua Marina** 84 Ebony Ct., Brooklyn, NY 11229, 718-646-9212

**Dr. John's Playground** Gerritsen Ave. and Avenue X, Brooklyn, NY 11229

**Marine Park** Avenue U and Burnett St., Brooklyn, NY 11234

**Salt Marsh Nature Center** 3302 Avenue U, Brooklyn, NY 11234, 718-421-2021

**Hendrick I. Lott House** 1940 E. 36th St., Brooklyn, NY 11234, 718-375-2681

**Lenape Playground** Avenue U at E. 37th St., Brooklyn, NY 11234

**Kings Plaza** Avenue U at Flatbush Ave., Brooklyn, NY 11234, 718-253-6842

**Dolly's Ices** Avenue U at E. 58th St., Brooklyn, NY 11234

## ADDENDUM

**Mill Basin Kosher Deli and Art Gallery** 5823 Avenue T, Brooklyn, NY 11234, 718-241-4910

# route summary

1. Begin at Gerritsen Ave. and Bartlett Pl. and go north on Gerritsen.
2. Turn left on Gotham Ave.
3. Turn right on Fane Ct.
4. Turn left on Everett Ave., then right on Joval Ct.
5. From the marina, walk east on Devon Ave. to Ebony Ct. and turn left.
6. From the Tamaqua Marina, go east on Channel Ave. to Gerritsen and turn left.
7. Turn right on Avenue X, then left on Burnett St.
8. Turn right on Avenue U.
9. Walk Marine Park's salt marsh trail on your right at E. 33rd St.
10. From the nature center, go right on Avenue U and then left on E. 36th St.
11. Turn right on Fillmore Ave., then turn right on E. 37th St. and proceed into Lenape Playground.
12. From the playground, go right on E. 38th St. Then go left on Avenue V.
13. Turn right on Flatbush Ave. and turn around just past Hendrickson Pl.
14. Turn right onto Avenue U.
15. Take the westbound B3 bus on Avenue U from E. 58th St. to the subway.

# addendum

16. From Avenue U, turn left on E. 58th and right at Avenue T.
17. Turn right on E. 63rd St.
18. Go left on Mayfair Dr. N. and right on E. 66th St.
19. From Bassett Ave. and E. 66th, get the B100 bus or walk back to Avenue U for the B3 bus.

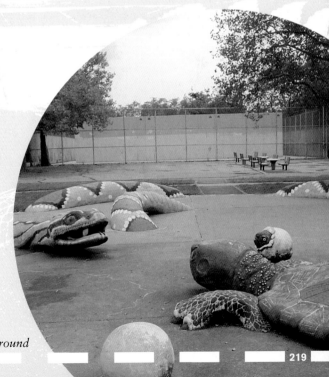

*Lenape Playground*

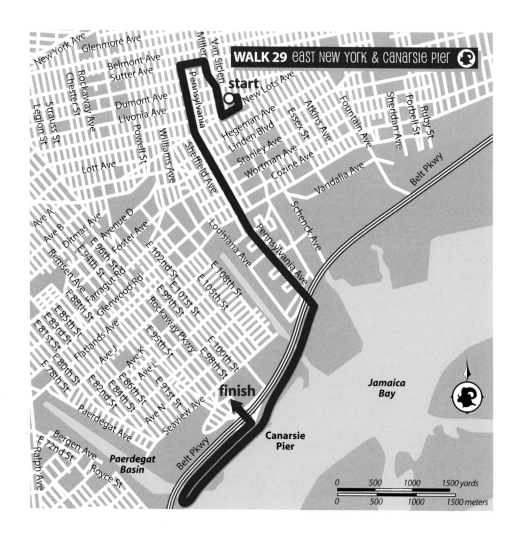

start

New Lots Ave

New York Ave
Glenmore Ave
Belmont Ave
Sutter Ave
Dumont Ave
Livonia Ave
Rockaway Ave
Chester St
Strauss St
Legion St
Lott Ave
Powell St
Williams Ave
Sheffield Ave
Pennsylvania
Miller
Van Siclen

Hegeman Ave
Linden Blvd
Stanley Ave
Wortman Ave
Cozine Ave
Essex St
Atkins Ave
Fountain Ave
Sheridan Ave
Forbell St
Ruby St

Vandalia Ave
Schenck Ave
Belt Pkwy

Louisiana Ave
Pennsylvania Ave

Ave A
Ave B
Ditmas Ave
Avenue D
Foster Ave
E 96th St
E 94th St
Remsen Ave
Farragut Rd
E 102nd St
E 101st St
E 99th St
E 108th St
E 105th St

E 88th St
E 85th St
E 83rd St
E 81st St
E 80th St
E 78th St
Glenwood Rd
Flatlands Ave
Ave J
Rockaway Pkwy
E 95th St
E 100th St
E 98th St

Ave K
Ave L
E 86th St
E 91st St
E 84th St
E 82nd St
Ave N
Seaview Ave

finish

Jamaica
Bay

Canarsie
Pier

Bergen Ave
E 72nd St
E Ralph Ave
Royce St
Paerdegat Ave
Paerdegat
Basin
Belt Pkwy

| 0 | 500 | 1000 | 1500 yards |
| 0 | 500 | 1000 | 1500 meters |

# 29 east New York and Canarsie Pier:
## The Stages of Urban Renewal

**BOUNDARIES:** Barbey St., Sutter Ave., Rockaway Pkwy., Belt Pkwy.
**DISTANCE:** Approx. 4 or 5¾ miles, depending on route chosen
**SUBWAY:** 3 to Van Siclen Ave.

In 1835, a Connecticut businessman named John Pitkin bought up land in the eastern reaches of Brooklyn with plans to create a city to rival Manhattan: East New York. An economic bulwark and employer of most residents of the community would be Pitkin's shoe factory. His dreams were dashed, however, by the so-called Panic of 1837, which forced Pitkin to give up much of the land and relocate farther east, in Queens. A worse fate was to befall East New York in the next century. It was among the hardest hit of New York City neighborhoods by drugs, crime, and poverty from the late 1960s into the '90s. At one point East New York ignominiously led the city in murders. But urban renewal eventually took hold, driven largely by church and civic groups. Though not without its struggles, it's a resurgent neighborhood today. This semi-adventurous walk tours urban renewal at various stages and concludes with a stroll along Jamaica Bay to Canarsie.

- From the subway, walk east on Livonia Ave. to Schenck Ave. Murals and gardens have been key elements of neighborhood improvement, involving citizens at a hands-on level. The New Vision community garden is on your near left, and across Schenck a mural tells the history of East New York. Another community garden, this one tended by students, is across Livonia from New Vision. Participating youth gain job skills and an agriculture education growing produce sold at the local farmers' market.

- Go one more block east on Livonia, past the playground, and turn right on Barbey St. The farmers' market is held on the grounds to your left every Saturday from June to November. The next avenue is New Lots, a name sometimes used for this part of East New York. The appellation originated in the 1600s when Dutch farmers moved into the area from the "old lots" that had already been cultivated to the west. Some of those Dutch families who first settled the area are buried in the ancient cemetery before you, which includes a Van Siclen plot.

- Turn right on New Lots Ave. Dutch farmers built this landmark church, New Lots Reformed, in 1823. They used oak trees felled by an 1821 hurricane for lumber and secured the building joints with wooden pegs. The community's first school was erected across the street, where the library is now. As you approach Schenck, look on your right for another colorful mural, this one depicting sociopolitical issues of concern to residents.

- Stay on New Lots to Miller Ave., then turn right. At Dumont St., walk through Martin Luther King Jr. Park, the only public park in all five boroughs named for Dr. King. The mural on the comfort station celebrates both white and black heroes of the fight for racial equality.

- Walk past the lawn of boulders and exit the park at its northwest corner, Blake Ave. and Bradford St., and go to your right on Bradford. There's another community garden on your left, but this block reverberates with the past. It's one of the few relatively untouched by the late-20th-century blight or the subsequent reconstruction.

- Turn left and walk on Sutter Ave. P.S. 149 at Wyona St. was built in 1905 and more recently renamed the Danny Kaye School, after one of its famous alumni.

- Turn left on Pennsylvania Ave., aka Granville Payne Ave. In the early 1900s the East New York area was home to many Jewish immigrants (like Danny Kaye's family), but few indications of that heritage remain. One can be found up high on the front of Mount Moriah church on your left: a Star of David, engraved on what must have been a synagogue. Thomas Jefferson High School, which you'll soon pass on your right, was once an academic powerhouse, but now comprises four separate schools (specializing in health professions, performing arts, firefighting, and African-American studies)—a tactic that has been applied to underperforming schools citywide.

- Take Pennsylvania Ave. all the way to the water. You can refuel during this long stretch at the Galaxy Diner, near Linden Blvd. At Flatlands Ave. you enter Starrett City (recently rechristened Spring Creek Towers), the country's largest federally subsidized housing complex, encompassing 46 buildings and 20,000 residents over 153 acres. It was conceived not so much as urban renewal as an experiment in preventing urban decline and forcing integration.  When it opened in the 1970s, those on public assistance were not allowed and just 30 percent of the units were available to blacks—an attempt to avert "white flight" from the area. But lawsuits and a dearth of white applicants led to abolition of the quotas. It's still a middle-income, diverse community.

- At Seaview Ave., keep going straight on Pennsylvania, crossing (carefully!) exit lanes for the Belt Pkwy. Another important cleanup is going on at the end of the avenue, where a Superfund site is gradually coming back to life. The decontaminated Pennsylvania Avenue Landfill is growing grass and trees—and eventually wildflowers and shrubbery—on what is envisioned to be a hillside park overlooking the bay. When you're in front of the landfill, turn right onto the Shore Parkway Bike Route. Jamaica Bay will come into view when you reach a bridge in about a ½ mile. You can see the Empire State Building (a good 15 miles yonder) to your right and the much closer Kennedy Airport in Queens to your left.

- The path will lead you right onto Canarsie Pier, which is part of the Gateway National Recreation Area. Fishermen used to make a living off oysters and clams from these waters, but the fishing here is now purely recreational. In the late 1800s, this was the transfer point between railroad and boat for New Yorkers headed for a beach vacation in the Rockaways. The wooden pier became the concrete structure it is now when the highway was built in the mid-20th century. The walk ends at this scenic spot, unless you opt for the addendum detailed below.

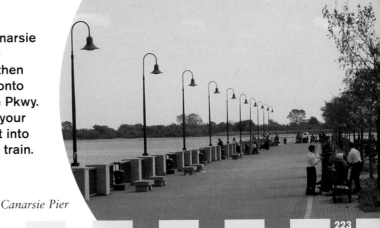

- To reach the subway from Canarsie Pier, follow the sidewalk halfway around the traffic circle, then walk through the underpass onto Rockaway Pkwy. Cross Shore Pkwy. and look for the bus stop on your right. The B42 takes you right into the Canarsie station for the L train.

*Canarsie Pier*

## DUTCH TREATS

Into the second half of the 20th century, more than 30 old Dutch farmhouses were still standing in Brooklyn. Only 14 are left—and one of those, the Jan Martense Schenck House (1676), is an indoor exhibition at the Brooklyn Museum, where it was reassembled in its entirety.

The oldest house in Brooklyn, in New York City, and maybe in New York State, is Pieter Claesen Wyckoff's. Built around 1652, it now operates as the Wyckoff Farmhouse Museum (Clarendon Rd. at Ralph Ave., 718-629-5400), complete with period objects and furnishings and a working farm. Though it's located beside a four-way intersection, it may be the country's most overlooked historical treasure, as no subway is nearby and the area (at the border of East Flatbush and Canarsie) is little

traveled except by people who live there. But the property is beautifully preserved and presents a vivid history lesson.

Several of the extant farmhouses (most privately owned) are situated in and around the Flatlands neighborhood of southeastern Brooklyn, inaccessible by subway and too spread out to tour on foot. The Van Nuyse-Coe House (1806) is at 1128-30 E. 34th St., right off Flatbush Ave., and the Stoothoff-Baxter-Kouwenhoven House is at 1640 E. 48th. The latter, a city landmark whose oldest wing dates to 1747, is located off Avenue N, close to a 1797 house at 1587 E. 53rd that has been severely modified. The Elias Hubbard Ryder House, at 1926 E. 28th, is an early-19th-century throwback in Midwood, where new mansions are more common.

Once Jewish and Italian, Canarsie is now predominantly Caribbean. Per residents' recreational preferences, a cricket field is being constructed as part of an upgrade of Canarsie Park, which sprawls over 132 acres west of the pier. Canarsie also contains four pre-1880 churches.

Addendum:

- From the pier, continue west on the bike path (look for access between the restrooms and the traffic circle). About ¾ mile from Canarsie Pier, you'll find yourself above Paerdegat Basin, with marinas, yacht clubs, and the volunteer-run Sebago Canoe Club, which offers free kayaking. If you want to go down to the small beaches of Jamaica Bay to your left, trails through the grass have been forged by previous explorers.

● To finish your walk, take the Belt Pkwy. path back to the pier and follow the directions on page 223 for the subway.

## POINTS OF INTEREST

**New Vision** Schenck and Livonia Aves., Brooklyn, NY 11207

**Martin Luther King Jr. Park** Dumont Ave. between Miller Ave. and Bradford St., Brooklyn, NY 11207

**Galaxy Diner** 805 Pennsylvania Ave., Brooklyn, NY 11207, 718-272-2660

**Canarsie Pier** Rockaway and Belt Pkwys., Brooklyn, NY 11236, 718-763-2202

## ADDENDUM

**Sebago Canoe Club** 1400 Paerdegat Ave. N., Brooklyn, NY 11236, 718-241-3683

## ROUTE SUMMARY

1. Walk east on Livonia Ave. from the subway at Van Siclen Ave.
2. Turn right on Barbey St.
3. Turn right on New Lots Ave.
4. Turn right on Miller Ave. and walk through Martin Luther King Jr. Park. Exit the park at Blake and Bradford and turn right on Bradford.
5. Go left on Sutter Ave.
6. Turn left on Pennsylvania Ave.
7. Cross Seaview Ave. and the Belt Pkwy. and go to your right onto the bike path to reach Canarsie Pier.
8. From the pier, cross a traffic circle and Shore Pkwy. onto Rockaway Pkwy., where you take the B42 bus to the L train.

## ADDENDUM

9. From Canarsie Pier, continue west on the bike path to the bridge over Paerdegat Basin and Jamaica Bay.
10. Turn around and go back to the pier, where you cross a traffic circle and Shore Pkwy. to get onto Rockaway Pkwy. for the B42 bus to the L train.

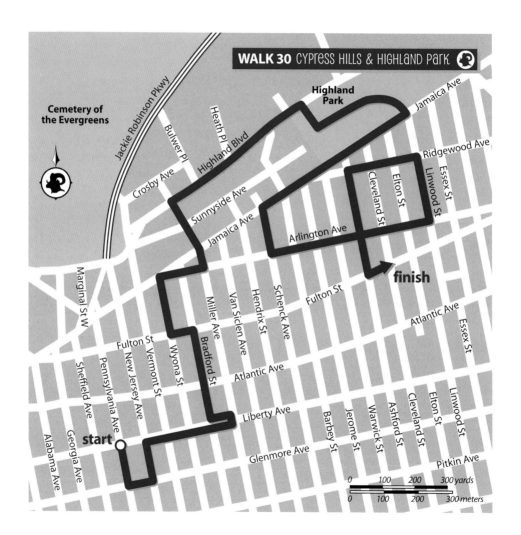

Cemetery of
the Evergreens

Highland
Park

Jackie Robinson Pkwy

Jamaica Ave

Ridgewood Ave

Essex St

Linwood St

Elton St

Cleveland St

Heath Pl

Bulwer Pl

Highland Blvd

Crosby Ave

Sunnyside Ave

Jamaica Ave

Arlington Ave

**finish**

Marginal St W

Miller Ave

Van Siclen Ave

Hendrix St

Schenck Ave

Fulton St

Atlantic Ave

Essex St

Fulton St

Vermont St

Wyona St

Bradford St

Atlantic Ave

Liberty Ave

**start**

Sheffield Ave

Pennsylvania Ave

New Jersey Ave

Georgia Ave

Alabama Ave

Glenmore Ave

Barbey St

Jerome St

Warwick St

Ashford St

Cleveland St

Elton St

Linwood St

Pitkin Ave

0    100    200    300 yards

0    100    200    300 meters

# 30 CYPRESS HILLS AND HIGHLAND PARK: ASTRIDE THE BORDER WITH QUEENS

**BOUNDARIES:** **Pennsylvania Ave., Highland Blvd., Linwood St., Glenmore Ave.**
**DISTANCE:** **Approx. 3 miles**
**SUBWAY:** **C to Liberty Ave.**

"Only the Dead Know Brooklyn," goes the title of a short story by Thomas Wolfe. He lived way over west in Cobble Hill, but the aphorism could apply to the easternmost nook of Brooklyn, where about 20 cemeteries straddle the border with Queens (including the one named Cypress Hills, NYC's only federal cemetery). In addition, there's a large city park half in Brooklyn, half in Queens—Highland Park, a name also used for the section of the Cypress Hills neighborhood nearest the park. Cypress Hills itself is sometimes considered a subcommunity of East New York. It was first regularly trafficked by horseracing fans going to Union Course, a track that opened just over the Queens line in 1821. Starting in the 1860s, it was part of a German belt that stretched across Brooklyn from Williamsburg. But most of Cypress Hills' growth into the neighborhood we know today took place around the turn of the century, when it developed as a suburb after John Pitkin's plan to turn East New York into a large city failed to materialize.

● Begin with a snippet of East New York. From the subway station, walk south on Pennsylvania/Granville Payne Ave. It's hard to miss the onion domes of Holy Trinity Russian Orthodox Church (1835) at Glenmore Ave., where you turn left. Another left onto New Jersey Ave. brings you to the *Kirche* for those early German residents, who named it St. Johannes. Built in 1885, it has since converted to Grace Baptist, but the original name in German is engraved on the façade.

● Turn right on Liberty Ave. On your right at Miller Ave. stands a castle without a dominion. This vacated Romanesque wonder is a twin of the landmark 68th Precinct Station House and Stable in Sunset Park, designed by the same architect in the same year (1892).

● Turn around and take Liberty back to Bradford St., where you turn right. Cross Atlantic Ave., the dividing line between East New York and Cypress Hills. Both communities were absorbed by the town of New Lots when it spun off in 1852 from Flatbush. The black-and-white apartment house on your right was erected in 1873 as New Lots Town Hall.

● Go left on Fulton St., followed by a right on Wyona St. At the end of Wyona, Jamaica and Arlington Aves. meet. Go to the right on Arlington. Then turn left on Miller Ave. and climb! You can carbo-load for the hike at D 'n' N Pizzeria just off Miller to your right at Jamaica. Up you go on Miller to Highland Blvd., which sits high on land created by the terminal moraine, a pileup of rock and soil left tens of thousands of years ago when glaciers receded. Go right on Highland—because of the views, this was prime real estate, as you can tell from the lavish homes. On your left after Heath Pl., #279 is one of the older ones, constructed in 1900.

● At Robert St., go down the staircase on your right. This takes you into Brooklyn's share of Highland Park. At the bottom of the 100-odd steps, turn left on the path. You'll be looking down on tennis courts to your right. Turn right on either of the two paths that lead you between the fields—they join up for a short stretch toward the bottom. When they rediverge, go left and follow the path past a playground to Linwood St. and Jamaica Ave.

● Turn right on Jamaica. The house at #494, across from the playground, is a Dutch farmhouse from the first half of the 19th century, possibly earlier. It was apparently owned by the Stoothoffs, one of the original farm families in the area.

● Proceeding on Jamaica, shift your gaze across the street to *Dawn of Glory,* a symbolic monument to World War I casualties. In the park on the next block is a children's garden. When you're past the park, watch on your right for Schenck Ct. Remember that the city of Brooklyn made a street grid out of land originally divided into farms, but some parcels, like this one, eluded the standardization.

● Go down Schenck Ave. and across Jamaica Ave. On your left at the next corner, the former Trinity Episcopal Church was designed in 1886 by Richard M. Upjohn, son of the architect of the more famous Trinity Church on Wall St. Stay on Schenck only to see the first house on the left across Arlington Ave. It makes a palatial trio with the matching manses at #124 and #130 on Arlington, all built around 1910.

- As you head east on Arlington, dip down Barbey St. to your left for the Lutheran Church of the Transformation, erected around 1909.

- Resume walking east on Arlington. Two lofty but disparate residences face each other across Jerome St. on your right: Classical versus a melange of brick, green shingle, and onion dome. At Warwick St. you'll find one of Brooklyn's earliest public libraries, opened in 1906 to serve the entire "East Branch" of Brooklyn (as the building still says). Ezra Jack Keats, the beloved author of such picture books as *The Snowy Day* and *A Whistle for Willie,* spent many hours reading in this library when he was growing up in East New York. It still has a charming old-fashioned interior.

- Turn left on Linwood. P.S. 108, on your left, is a city landmark and listed on the National Register of Historic Places for its age (built in 1895) and Romanesque styling.

- Go left on Ridgewood Ave. Before turning left on Ashford St., have a look at the Ridgewood side of 18 Ashford St.—asymmetrically busy with bay and gingerbread windows. The house is calmer in front, though all of this Victorian classic from 1904 has been injudiciously sheathed in contemporary siding. Farther down Ashford is a circa-1885 home at #68.

- Take Ashford to Fulton and go left for the J train at Cleveland St.

*Holy Trinity Russian Orthodox Church*

## POINTS OF INTEREST

**D 'n' N Pizzeria** 188 Jamaica Ave., Brooklyn, NY 11207, 718-235-3900

**Highland Park** Highland Blvd. to Jamaica Ave., Brooklyn, NY 11208

**Brooklyn Public Library–Arlington** 203 Arlington Ave., Brooklyn, NY 11207, 718-277-6105

## route summary

1. Starting at Liberty Ave., walk south on Pennsylvania Ave. Go left on Glenmore Ave. and then left on New Jersey Ave.

2. Turn right on Liberty to Miller Ave.

3. Turn around and turn right from Liberty onto Bradford St.

4. Turn left on Fulton St., right on Wyona St., right on Arlington Ave., left on Miller, and finally right on Highland Blvd.

5. At Robert St., walk down the staircase and through Highland Park.

6. Turn right on Jamaica Ave. at Linwood St.

7. Walk south on Schenck Ave.

8. Turn left on Arlington Ave. and dip down Barbey St.

9. Resume walking on Arlington and turn left on Linwood.

10. Turn left on Ridgewood Ave. and left on Ashford St.

11. Go left on Fulton St. to the subway at Cleveland St.

# APPENDIX 1: WALKS BY THEME

## arts and Culture

**Manhattan Bridge and Ferry District** (Walk 2)
**Dumbo and Vinegar Hill** (Walk 3)
**Carroll Gardens and Gowanus** (Walk 7)
**Red Hook** (Walk 8)
**Prospect Heights** (Walk 11)
**Fort Greene** (Walk 16)
**Clinton Hill** (Walk 17)
**Williamsburg** (Walk 19)

## Houses and Churches

**Brooklyn Heights** (Walk 5)
**Boerum Hill and Cobble Hill** (Walk 6)
**Carroll Gardens and Gowanus** (Walk 7)
**Park Slope** (Walk 9)
**Prospect Heights** (Walk 11)
**Flatbush and Midwood** (Walk 13)
**Crown Heights** (Walk 14)
**Bedford-Stuyvesant** (Walk 15)
**Fort Greene** (Walk 16)
**Clinton Hill** (Walk 17)
**Bushwick** (Walk 18)
**Greenpoint** (Walk 20)
**Bay Ridge** (Walk 23)
**Cypress Hills and Highland Park** (Walk 30)

## Ethnic Heritage

**Carroll Gardens and Gowanus** (Walk 7)
**Flatbush and Midwood** (Walk 13)
**Crown Heights** (Walk 14)
**Bedford-Stuyvesant** (Walk 15)
**Fort Greene** (Walk 16)
**Williamsburg** (Walk 19)
**Greenpoint** (Walk 20)
**Sunset Park** (Walk 22)
**Fort Hamilton to Bensonhurst** (Walk 24)
**Coney Island and Brighton Beach** (Walk 26)

## History

**Manhattan Bridge and Ferry District** (Walk 2)
**Dumbo and Vinegar Hill** (Walk 3)
**Downtown** (Walk 4)
**Red Hook** (Walk 8)
**Prospect Park** (Walk 10)
**Around Prospect Park** (Walk 12)
**Flatbush and Midwood** (Walk 13)
**Fort Greene** (Walk 16)
**Williamsburg** (Walk 19)
**The Green-Wood Cemetery** (Walk 21)
**Fort Hamilton to Bensonhurst** (Walk 24)
**Gravesend** (Walk 25)

## NeIGHBorHOODS IN TranSITION

**Dumbo and Vinegar Hill** (Walk 3)
**Downtown** (Walk 4)
**Carroll Gardens and Gowanus** (Walk 7)
**Red Hook** (Walk 8)
**Bushwick** (Walk 18)
**Williamsburg** (Walk 19)
**Greenpoint** (Walk 20)
**East New York and Canarsie Pier** (Walk 29)

## SHOPPING

**Manhattan Bridge and Ferry District** (Walk 2)
**Dumbo and Vinegar Hill** (Walk 3)
**Downtown** (Walk 4)
**Brooklyn Heights** (Walk 5)
**Boerum Hill and Cobble Hill** (Walk 6)
**Park Slope** (Walk 9)
**Fort Greene** (Walk 16)
**Greenpoint** (Walk 20)

## waTerFronT

**Brooklyn Bridge and Brooklyn Heights Promenade** (Walk 1)
**Manhattan Bridge and Ferry District** (Walk 2)
**Carroll Gardens and Gowanus** (Walk 7)
**Red Hook** (Walk 8)
**Williamsburg** (Walk 19)
**Bay Ridge** (Walk 23)
**Fort Hamilton to Bensonhurst** (Walk 24)
**Coney Island and Brighton Beach** (Walk 26)
**Manhattan Beach and Sheepshead Bay** (Walk 27)
**Marine Park, Gerritsen Beach, and Mill Basin** (Walk 28)
**East New York and Canarsie Pier** (Walk 29)

# APPENDIX 2: POINTS OF INTEREST

## FOOD AND DRINK

**Alex Aguinaga Restaurant** 214 Knickerbocker Ave., Brooklyn, NY 11237, 718-497-2828

**Alma** 187 Columbia St., Brooklyn, NY 11231, 718-643-5400

**Baked** 359 Van Brunt St., Brooklyn, NY 11231, 718-222-0345

**Bake Ridge Bagels** 9417 3rd Ave., Brooklyn, NY 11209, 718-680-6353

**Ballybunion** 9510 3rd Ave., Brooklyn, NY 11209, 718-833-2801

**Barcade** 388 Union Ave., Brooklyn, NY 11211, 718-302-6464

**The Blue Pig** 60 Henry St., Brooklyn, NY 11201, 718-596-6301

**Brooklyn Ice Cream Factory** Fulton Ferry Landing, Brooklyn, NY 11201, 718-246-3963

**Brooklyn Inn** 138 Bergen St., Brooklyn, NY 11217, 718-625-9741

**Bubby's** 1 Main St., Brooklyn, NY 11201, 718-222-0666

**Cafe Kai** 151 Smith St., Brooklyn, NY 11201, 718-596-3466

**Canal Bar** 270 3rd Ave., Brooklyn, NY 11215, 718-246-0011

**The Chocolate Room** 86 5th Ave., Brooklyn, NY 11217, 718-783-2900

**Christie's Jamaican Patties** 387 Flatbush Ave., Brooklyn, NY 11238, 718-636-9746

**Cocoa Bar** 228 7th Ave., Brooklyn, NY 11215, 718-499-4080

**Cranberry's** 48 Henry St., Brooklyn, NY 11201, 718-624-3500

**Diner** 85 Broadway, Brooklyn, NY 11211, 718-486-3077

**D 'n' N Pizzeria** 188 Jamaica Ave., Brooklyn, NY 11207, 718-235-3900

**Dolly's Ices** Avenue U at E. 58th St., Brooklyn, NY 11234

**Downtown Atlantic** 364 Atlantic Ave., Brooklyn, NY 11217, 718-852-9945

**The Farm on Adderley** 1108 Cortelyou Rd., Brooklyn, NY 11218, 718-287-3101

**Farrell's** 215 Prospect Park W., Brooklyn, NY 11215, 718-788-8779

**Ferdinando's** 151 Union St., Brooklyn, NY 11231, 718-855-1545

**Food 4 Thought** 445 Marcus Garvey Blvd., Brooklyn, NY 11216, 718-443-4160

**Galaxy Diner** 805 Pennsylvania Ave., Brooklyn, NY 11207, 718-272-2660

**Grimaldi's** 19 Old Fulton St., Brooklyn, NY 11201, 718-858-4300

**Habana Outpost** 757 Fulton St., Brooklyn, NY 11217, 718-858-9500

**Heru's Juice Bar** 111 Kingston Ave., Brooklyn, NY 11213, 718-756-9807

**International Restaurant** 4408 5th Ave., Brooklyn, NY 11220, 718-438-2009

**Jacques Torres Chocolate** 66 Water St., Brooklyn, NY 11201, 718-875-9772

**Junior's** Flatbush and DeKalb Aves., Brooklyn, NY 11201, 718-852-5257

**K&B Carib Kitchen** 268 Kingston Ave., Brooklyn, NY 11213, 718-363-1118

**Kashkar Café** 1141 Brighton Beach Ave., Brooklyn, NY 11235, 718-743-3832

**Lassen & Hennigs** 114 Montague St., Brooklyn, NY 11201, 718-875-6272

**Liberty Heights Tap Room** 34 Van Dyke St., Brooklyn, NY 11231, 718-246-8050

**Marlow & Sons** 81 Broadway, Brooklyn, NY 11211, 718-384-1441

**M&I International** 249 Brighton Beach Ave., Brooklyn, NY 11235, 718-615-1011

**Masal Cafe** 1901 Emmons Ave., Brooklyn, NY 11235, 718-891-7090

**Mike's Coffee Shop** 328 DeKalb Ave., Brooklyn, NY 11205, 718-857-1462

**Mike's International** 552 Flatbush Ave., Brooklyn, NY 11225, 718-856-7034

**Mill Basin Kosher Deli and Art Gallery** 5823 Avenue T, Brooklyn, NY 11234, 718-241-4910

**Nathan's** Surf and Stillwell Aves., Brooklyn, NY 11224, 718-946-2202

**Nuccio's** 261 Avenue U, Brooklyn, NY 11223, 718-449-3035

**Old Pioneer Bar** 318 Van Brunt St., Brooklyn, NY 11231, 718-624-0700

**Old Poland** 190 Nassau Ave., Brooklyn, NY 11222, 718-349-7775

**Oslo Coffee Company** 133 Roebling St., Brooklyn, NY 11211, 718-782-0332

**Ozzie's** 57 7th Ave., Brooklyn, NY 11215, 718-398-6695

**Pak Sweets & Grill** 998 Coney Island Ave., Brooklyn, NY 11230, 718-421-0505

**Pedro's Spanish American Restaurant** 73 Jay St., Brooklyn, NY 11201, 718-625-0031

**Peter Luger** 178 Broadway, Brooklyn, NY 11211, 718-387-7400

**Peter Pan Donut & Pastry Shop** 727 Manhattan Ave., Brooklyn, NY 11222, 718-383-9442

**Pete's Downtown** 2 Water St., Brooklyn, NY 11201, 718-858-3510

**P.J. Hanley's** 449 Court St., Brooklyn, NY 11231, 718-834-8223

**Primorski** 282 Brighton Beach Ave., Brooklyn, NY 11235, 718-891-3111

**Randazzo's** 2017 Emmons Ave., Brooklyn, NY 11235, 718-615-0010

**Red Hook Bait & Tackle Shop Fishing Club** 320 Van Brunt St., Brooklyn, NY 11231, 718-797-4892

**Retreat** 147 Front St., Brooklyn, NY 11201, 718-797-2322

**Ruthies** 96 DeKalb Ave., Brooklyn, NY 11201, 718-246-5189

**Schnäck** 122 Union St., Brooklyn, NY 11231, 718-855-2879

**Steve's Authentic Key Lime Pies** Pier 41/204 Van Dyke St., Brooklyn, NY 11231, 718-858-5333

**Sunny's** 253 Conover St., Brooklyn, NY 11231, 718-625-8211

**Superfine** 126 Front St., Brooklyn, NY 11201, 718-243-9005

**Tamaqua Marina** 84 Ebony Ct., Brooklyn, NY 11229, 718-646-9212

**West End Bakery** 8517 18th Ave., Brooklyn, NY 11214, 718-259-0777

# entertainment and nightlife

**Bargemusic** Fulton Ferry Landing, Brooklyn, NY 11201, 718-624-4061/2083
**Brooklyn Academy of Music** 30 Lafayette Ave., Brooklyn, NY 11217, 718-636-4100
**Brooklyn Lyceum** 227 4th Ave., Brooklyn, NY 11215, 866-GOWANUS
**Europa Night Club** 98 Meserole Ave., Brooklyn, NY 11222, 718-383-5723
**Heights Players** 26 Willow Pl., Brooklyn, NY 11201, 718-237-2752
**Issue Project Room** 400 Carroll St., Brooklyn, NY 11231, 718-330-0313
**Sackett Group** 126 St. Felix St., Brooklyn, NY 11217, 718-638-7104
**Sideshows by the Seashore** 3006 W. 12th St., Brooklyn, NY 11224, 718-372-5159
**St. Ann's Warehouse** 38 Water St., Brooklyn, NY 11201, 718-858-2424
**Warsaw** Polish National Home, 261 Driggs Ave., Brooklyn, NY 11222, 718-387-0505

# museums and galleries

**Brooklyn Children's Museum** 145 Brooklyn Ave., Brooklyn, NY 11213, 718-735-4400
**Brooklyn Historical Society** 128 Pierrepont St., Brooklyn, NY 11201, 718-222-4111
**Brooklyn Museum** 200 Eastern Pkwy., Brooklyn, NY 11238, 718-638-5000
**City Reliquary** 370 Metropolitan Ave., Brooklyn, NY 11211, 718-782-4842
**Coney Island Museum** 1208 Surf Ave., Brooklyn, NY 11224, 718-372-5159
**Enrico Caruso Museum of America** 1942 E. 19th St., Brooklyn, NY 11229, 718-368-3993
**Fort Hamilton's Harbor Defense Museum** 230 Sheridan Loop, Brooklyn, NY 11252, 718-630-4349
**Front Street Galleries** 111 Front St., Brooklyn, NY 11201
**gallerythe.org** 343 Smith St., Brooklyn, NY 11231
**Jan Larsen Art** 63 Pearl St., Brooklyn, NY 11201, 718-797-2557
**Jewish Children's Museum** 792 Eastern Pkwy., Brooklyn, NY 11213, 718-467-0600
**Kentler International Drawing Space** 353 Van Brunt St., Brooklyn, NY 11231, 718-875-2098
**Lefferts Historic House** Prospect Park near Flatbush Ave. and Empire Blvd., Brooklyn, NY 11215, 718-789-2822
**Micro Museum** 123 Smith St., Brooklyn, NY 11201, 718-797-3116
**MoCADA** 80 Hanson Pl. (on S. Portland Ave.), Brooklyn, NY 11217, 718-230-0492
**New York Transit Museum** Boerum Pl. and Schermerhorn St., Brooklyn, NY 11201, 718-694-1600
**Old Stone House** J.J. Byrne Park, 3rd St. and 5th Ave., Brooklyn, NY 11215, 718-768-3195
**Photo Gallery of Williamsburg** 437 Grand St., Brooklyn, NY 11211, 718-782-3433

**powerHouse Arena** 37 Main St., Brooklyn, NY 11201, 718-666-3049

**RSA Diesel Gallery** 242 Van Brunt St., Brooklyn, NY 11231, 917-251-4070

**Smack Mellon** 92 Plymouth St., Brooklyn, NY 11201, 718-834-8761

**Spring** 126 Front St., Brooklyn, NY 11201, 718-222-1054

**Urban Glass** 57 Rockwell Pl., Brooklyn, NY 11217, 718-625-3685

**Waterfront Museum** 290 Conover St., Brooklyn, NY 11231, 718-624-4719

**Wyckoff Farmhouse Museum** Clarendon Rd. at Ralph Ave., Brooklyn, NY 11203, 718-629-5400

## eDucaTioNaL aND cuLTuraL ceNTers

**Audubon Center at the Boathouse** Prospect Park near Ocean Ave. and Lincoln Rd., Brooklyn, NY 11215, 718-287-3400

**Brooklyn Center for the Urban Environment** Tennis House, Prospect Park near 9th St., Brooklyn, NY 11215, 718-788-8500

**Brooklyn College** 2900 Bedford Ave., Brooklyn, NY 11210, 718-951-5000

**Brooklyn Information & Culture (BRIC)** 647 Fulton St., Brooklyn, NY 11217, 718-855-7882

**Brooklyn Public Library** Flatbush Ave. and Eastern Pkwy., Brooklyn, NY 11238, 718-230-2100

**Brooklyn Public Library–Arlington** 203 Arlington Ave., Brooklyn, NY 11207, 718-277-6105

**Brooklyn Public Library–Gerritsen Beach** 2808 Gerritsen Ave., Brooklyn, NY 11229, 718-368-1435

**Brooklyn Public Library–Walt Whitman** 93 St. Edwards St., Brooklyn, NY 11205, 718-935-0244

**Brooklyn Public Library–Williamsburgh** Division and Marcy Aves., Brooklyn, NY 11211, 718-302-3485

**Hunterfly Road Houses/Weeksville Heritage Center** 1698 Bergen St., Brooklyn, NY 11213, 718-756-5250

**Kingsborough Community College** 2001 Oriental Blvd., Brooklyn, NY 11235, 718-265-5343

**Magnolia Tree Earth Center** 677 Lafayette Ave., Brooklyn, NY 11216, 718-387-2116

**Pratt Institute** 200 Willoughby Ave., Brooklyn, NY 11205, 718-636-3600

**Salt Marsh Nature Center** 3302 Avenue U, Brooklyn, NY 11234, 718-421-2021

**Williamsburg Art & Historical Center** 135 Broadway, Brooklyn, NY 11211, 718-486-7372

## HisToric Houses aND BuiLDiNGs

**Akwaaba Mansion** 347 MacDonough St., Brooklyn, NY 11233, 718-455-5958

**Dime Savings Bank (Washington Mutual)** 9 DeKalb Ave., Brooklyn, NY 11201, 718-403-7900

**Erasmus Hall Academy** 911 Flatbush Ave., Brooklyn, NY 11226

**Green Point Savings Bank (North Fork Bank)** 807 Manhattan Ave., Brooklyn, NY 11222, 718-706-2901

**Hendrick I. Lott House** 1940 E. 36th St., Brooklyn, NY 11234, 718-375-2681

**Hubbard House** 2138 McDonald Ave., Brooklyn, NY 11223

**Johannes Van Nuyse House** 1041 E. 22nd St., Brooklyn, NY 11210

**Lady Moody's House** 27 Gravesend Neck Rd., Brooklyn, NY 11223

**Lefferts Historic House** Prospect Park near Flatbush Ave. and Empire Blvd., Brooklyn, NY 11215, 718-789-2822

**Litchfield Villa** Prospect Park W. and 5th St., Brooklyn, NY 11215, 718-965-8900

**Old Stone House** J.J. Byrne Park, 3rd St. and 5th Ave., Brooklyn, NY 11215, 718-768-3195

**Pieter Claesen Wyckoff House** Clarendon Rd. at Ralph Ave., Brooklyn, NY 11203, 718-629-5400

**Ryder-Van Cleef House** 38 Village Rd. N., Brooklyn, NY 11223

**South Brooklyn Savings Institution (Sovereign Bank)** 130 Court St., Brooklyn, NY 11201, 718-637-2205

**Williamsburgh Savings Bank** 1 Hanson Pl., Brooklyn, NY 11217

**Williamsburgh Savings Bank (HSBC)** 175 Broadway, Brooklyn, NY 11211

**Williamsburg Trust Company** S. 5th St. and S. 5th Pl., Brooklyn, NY 11211

**Wyckoff-Bennett Homestead** 1669 E. 22nd St., Brooklyn, NY 11229

## SHOPPING

**BookCourt** 163 Court St., Brooklyn, NY 11201, 718-875-3677

**Brownstone Books** 409 Lewis Ave., Brooklyn, NY 11233, 718-953-7328

**Fairway of Red Hook** 480–500 Van Brunt St., Brooklyn, NY 11231, 718-694-6868

**Fishs Eddy** 122 Montague St., Brooklyn, NY 11201, 718-797-3990

**Frankel's** 3924 3rd Ave., Brooklyn, NY 11232, 718-768-9788

**Halcyon** 57 Pearl St., Brooklyn, NY 11201, 718-260-9299

**Journey** 166 Water St., Brooklyn, NY 11201, 718-797-9277

**Kings Plaza** Avenue U at Flatbush Ave., Brooklyn, NY 11234, 718-253-6842

**Loopy Mango** 117 Front St., Brooklyn, NY 11201, 718-858-5930

**powerHouse Arena** 37 Main St., Brooklyn, NY 11201, 718-666-3049

**P.S. Bookshop** 145 Front St., Brooklyn, NY 11201, 718-222-3340

**Spoonbill & Sugartown Booksellers** 218 Bedford Ave., Brooklyn, NY 12111, 718-387-7322

**Spring** 126 Front St., Brooklyn, NY 11201, 718-222-1054

**Urban Glass** 57 Rockwell Pl., Brooklyn, NY 11217, 718-625-3685

# ParKS anD GarDens

**American Veterans Memorial Pier** 69th St. at Shore Rd., Brooklyn, NY 11209

**Asser Levy Park** W. 5th St. between Surf and Seaview Aves., Brooklyn, NY 11224

**Bath Beach Park** 17th Ave. and 17th Ct., Brooklyn, NY 11214

**Brooklyn Botanic Garden** 1000 Washington Ave., Brooklyn, NY 11225, 718-623-7200

**Brooklyn Bridge Park** Plymouth St. between Adams and Main Sts., Brooklyn, NY 11201, 718-802-0603

**Brower Park** Prospect Pl. between Brooklyn and Kingston Aves., Brooklyn, NY 11213

**Cadman Plaza Park** Tillary St. and Cadman Plaza, Brooklyn, NY 11201

**Canarsie Pier** Rockaway and Belt Pkwys., Brooklyn, NY 11236, 718-763-2202

**Carroll Park** Smith and President Sts., Brooklyn, NY 11231

**Cobble Hill Park** Clinton St. and Verandah Pl., Brooklyn, NY 11201

**Coffey Park** Richards and Verona Sts., Brooklyn, NY 11231

**Dr. John's Playground** Gerritsen Ave. and Avenue X, Brooklyn, NY 11229

**Dr. Ronald McNair Park** Eastern Pkwy. and Washington Ave., Brooklyn, NY 11225

**Dyker Beach Park** Bay 8th St. and Cropsey Ave., Brooklyn, NY 11228

**Empire-Fulton Ferry State Park** 6 New Dock St., Brooklyn, NY 11201, 718-858-4708

**Father Jerzy Popieluszko Square** Bedford and Nassau Aves., Brooklyn, NY 11222

**Fort Greene Park** Myrtle Ave. between St. Edwards St. and Washington Park, Brooklyn, NY 11217

**Fulton Park** Chauncey St. between Lewis and Stuyvesant Aves., Brooklyn, NY 11233

**Garden Pier** Conover and Beard Sts., Brooklyn, NY 11231

**Garibaldi Playground** 18th Ave. between 82nd and 83rd Sts., Brooklyn, NY 11214

**Grand Ferry Park** Grand St. off Kent Ave., Brooklyn, NY 11211

**Green Dome Garden** McCarren Park at N. 12th, Brooklyn, NY 11222

**Greene Garden** DeKalb Ave. between S. Portland Ave. and S. Elliott Pl., Brooklyn, NY 11217

**The Green-Wood Cemetery** 5th Ave. at 25th St., Brooklyn, NY 11232, 718-768-7300

**Harry Chapin Playground** Columbia Heights and Middagh St., Brooklyn, NY 11201

**Herbert Von King Park** Greene Ave. between Marcy and Tompkins Aves., Brooklyn, NY 11216

**Highland Park** Highland Blvd. to Jamaica Ave., Brooklyn, NY 11208

**Holocaust Memorial Park** Shore Blvd. and Emmons Ave., Brooklyn, NY 11235, 718-743-3636

**Hoyt Street Garden** Hoyt St. at Atlantic Ave., Brooklyn, NY 11217

**J.J. Byrne Park** 3rd St. and 5th Ave., Brooklyn, NY 11215

**John Paul Jones Park** 4th Ave. and 101st St., Brooklyn, NY 11209

**Justice Gilbert Ramirez Park** McKibbin and White Sts., Brooklyn, NY 11206

**Lady Moody Triangle** Van Sicklen St. between Avenue U and Village Rd. N., Brooklyn, NY 11223

**Lenape Playground** Avenue U at E. 37th St., Brooklyn, NY 11234

**Manhattan Beach Park** Oriental Blvd. between Ocean Ave. and Mackenzie St., Brooklyn, NY 11235

**Maria Hernandez Park** Irving Ave. between White and Starr Sts., Brooklyn, NY 11237

**Marine Park** Avenue U and Burnett St., Brooklyn, NY 11234

**Martin Luther King Jr. Park** Dumont Ave. between Miller Ave. and Bradford St., Brooklyn, NY 11207

**McCarren Park** Bedford Ave. and Bayard St., Brooklyn, NY 11222

**Milestone Park** 18th Ave. between 81st and 82nd Sts., Brooklyn, NY 11214

**Monsignor McGolrick Park** Driggs Ave. and Russell St., Brooklyn, NY 11222

**Mount Prospect Park** Eastern Pkwy. at Underhill Ave., Brooklyn, NY 11238

**Narrows Botanical Garden** Shore Rd. between Bay Ridge Ave. and 72nd St., Brooklyn, NY 11209

**New Vision** Schenck and Livonia Aves., Brooklyn, NY 11207

**North Pacific Playground** Pacific St. between 3rd Ave. and Nevins St., Brooklyn, NY 11217

**Parade Ground** Parkside to Caton Aves. at Coney Island Ave., Brooklyn, NY 11218, 718-438-3435

**Prospect Park** Grand Army Plaza, Brooklyn, NY 11215, 718-965-8951

**Red Hook Community Farm** Columbia and Sigourney Sts., Brooklyn, NY 11231

**Sunset Park** 5th to 7th Aves. between 41st and 44th Sts., Brooklyn, NY 11220

**Tilyou Playground** Brighton Beach Ave. between Brighton 11th and 13th Sts., Brooklyn, NY 11224

**Underwood Park** Washington and Lafayette Aves., Brooklyn, NY 11205

**Upper Van Voorhees Park** Hicks St. between Atlantic Ave. and Congress St., Brooklyn, NY 11201

**Valentino Pier** Coffey and Ferris Sts., Brooklyn, NY 11231

## Miscellaneous

**Astroland Amusement Park** Coney Island Boardwalk at W. 10th St., Brooklyn, NY 11224, 718-265-2100

**Deno's Amusement Park** Coney Island Boardwalk at W. 12th St., Brooklyn, NY 11224, 718-372-2592

**Faith Camii mosque** 5911 8th Ave., Brooklyn, NY 11220, 718-438-6919

**Fort Hamilton** 101st St. and Fort Hamilton Pkwy., Brooklyn, NY 11252, 718-630-4101

**Gowanus Dredgers** 2nd St. at Gowanus Canal, Brooklyn, NY 11231, 718-243-0849

**New Foundry New York** 220 India St., Brooklyn, NY 11222, 718-389-8172

**New York Aquarium** W. 8th St. and Surf Ave., Brooklyn, NY 11224, 718-265-FISH

**Prospect Park Zoo** Near Flatbush Ave. and Empire Blvd., Brooklyn, NY 11215, 718-399-7339

**Sebago Canoe Club** 1400 Paerdegat Ave. N., Brooklyn, NY 11236, 718-241-3683

# INDEX

*Italicized* page numbers indicate photographs.

# about the author

Adrienne Onofri is a native New Yorker. As a travel writer, she has covered destinations from the Caribbean to Asia but had never written so extensively about her hometown until this book. She is a licensed NYC sightseeing guide, specializing in customized walking tours and cultural/recreational recommendations for visitors. Adrienne has been a staff editor at several travel trade publications and is currently a freelance editor for national consumer magazines. She is also a theater writer and member of the Drama Desk. She received a bachelor's degree in journalism from Northwestern University and a master's degree from Pace University, where she has taught writing. *Walking Brooklyn* is her first book.

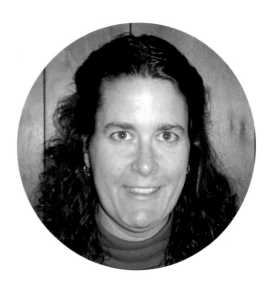

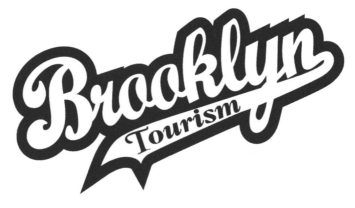

Brooklyn Tourism promotes Brooklyn's diversity, unique attractions, and cultural institutions. A non-profit initiative of Brooklyn Borough President Marty Markowitz, it operates the Brooklyn Tourism & Visitors Center in Brooklyn Borough Hall. Visit the center at 209 Joralemon Street, between Court Street and Adams Street or see www.visitbrooklyn.org for more information on exploring New York City's largest, hippest borough.